HOMECARE:
The Best!

D0170000

HOMECARE:
The Best!

How to Get it, Give it, and Live with It

Jo Whatley Cheatham

A practical guide for those who need, or anticipate needing homecare, their advocates, and their caregivers

ProSo Press

Manufactured in the United States of America
Library of Congress Catalog Card Number: 99-74180
ISBN: 0-9670880-0-3
Cover design: Pearl & Associates

Disclaimer:
A text covering the topic of homecare could not be written without mention of legal, financial, and psychological aspects of the subject. Information contained in this volume that refers to any profession connected with the homecare process is not to be construed as legal, financial, or psychological advice. If the reader should need advice on a particular subject, an expert in that field should be consulted.

Material contained in this book has been carefully researched and edited. Typographical errors and content errors may be found within the text, but they, of course, are not intended to mislead or confuse the reader.

The purpose of this book is to educate and inform. The author and ProSo Press do not accept any implied or real responsibility or liability for loss or damage, which may be claimed by any reader of this book.

If you do not wish to be bound by the above, you may return this book to the publisher for a full refund.

The publisher acknowledges the following as registered trademarks: Rolodex, Evian, Via-TV, Stouffer's, Energizer, and Polaroid.

ProSo Press
3190 North Atlantic Avenue, #102
Cocoa Beach, FL 32931
www.problemsolvers8.xtcom.com

To my mother, better known as "Granny,"
To my husband, Walter,
And to my three daughters,
Sonja, Sarina, and Misty–
my guides through life.

Contents

Section III

The Caregiver or Homeworker:
Friend/Family Member/Professional

Appendix A

Appendix B

Appendix C

Appendix D

Appendix E

Index

From the Author

I've been hit in the head with a three-legged cane. I've gone hoarse trying to convince a client that Vanna was in the TV, that she couldn't sit down to dinner with us. I've cooked six eggs in a row, attempting to get a "soft-boiled" egg perfect. I've sat in a dimly lit condo lobby at 2:00 A.M., because my client wanted to "see who's out there." I've counted the same $287 thirty times and been summoned to count it *one more time*. I've listened to a client brag to her friends, "Jo is at my beck and call, she does what I tell her," and I've been run ragged for twenty-hour stretches by clients who were convinced I was the Energizer Bunny.

On the other hand, I've had the privilege of working for some of the sweetest people on earth. I've received respect and appreciation from most of my clients, their friends, and family members. I've gained precious perspective about the caregiver's role. I've learned patience from both clients and co-workers, and I've been exposed to people, places, and things that have helped me to grow in all ways. And from every client I have worked for, I have gained insights into, and understanding of, the process of aging and the desire for independence that is innate in the majority of us.

For all my experiences, good and bad, I have learned to be thankful. Even the blow to my head from that cane taught me something: always be alert, always be aware, a tragedy can happen in a split second. What made me sit up and take notice was not the lump on my head, but my client's thin skin that tore when I grabbed her arm. She was ninety-seven. I learned not to underestimate the strength that can erupt from frustration and suppressed anger.

The first time I remember thinking in terms of age, loneliness, and dependency, I was ten years old. With my mother I made the trip to a small country nursing home to see Aunt Sally, my great-aunt.

A stale ammonia smell wafted along the long, cold hallway. I watched from the open doorway as my mother joined Aunt Sally, who sat on the edge of a small bed by an uncurtained window. My great-aunt's white fluff of hair and cornflower blue eyes gave her an angelic look. Myriad wrinkles above her glasses and in her pale cheeks gave her face the look of a mussed sheet. I didn't really know Aunt Sally, and I didn't realize that I was taking on and feeling her vulnerability. I just knew that I instantly loved her.

I wanted to take Aunt Sally home with us and wondered aloud to my mother why we couldn't. I don't remember what my mother told me, but I do remember that I couldn't comprehend why Aunt Sally would live in that place when she had a family.

Over the years, I have learned of many reasons why some people have to live away from their own homes, away from friends and relatives. And no one can judge another for decisions made. As Howie Mandel has said, "Well, what would *you* do?"

Indeed, what will we do when we face the fact that a friend or relative needs care—care that we are unable to give? And how will we accept needing care, when and if our time comes? I think about these questions, and the only way I come close to finding answers is by slipping off my shoes and walking for a while in someone else's. That exercise leaves me with one of several reactions: I weep, I turn rigid with anger, or I anguish in helpless frustration.

Over the years, I have seen and felt the tears, anger, and frustration of my clients, their family members, and their devoted friends. Already suffering physical, emotional, and sometimes mental pain from illness, disability, frailty, or loneliness, those clients suffered in their search for a homeworker as well. Every situation I encountered was heartwrenching in some respect.

Not only have I witnessed the havoc of setting up homecare in households where I worked, but I have also encountered difficulties as I set up and provided care for several relatives in home settings and for my husband in our own home.

Asthma, bronchitis, cancer, sciatica and back surgery, emphysema, coma, heart disease, chronic pain, diabetes, stroke, malabsorption—the list goes on— people I love, people I know well.

More than once I have attempted to leave the field of home healthcare and find my way in another profession where I wouldn't feel the pain, witness the vulnerability, or suffer the emotional exhaustion that comes with caregiving. But I stayed. At least, I kept coming back, and I finally figured out why. There is a unique feeling I get from seeing a person through the uneasiness of the night, the sunshine of hope, the twilight of life. I was with my grandmother when she died. I had my back turned for just a moment when, three feet away, a client of the most mild manner passed on without a sound. I held my father's hand and told him, "It's all right, you can go now," and he did. I like to think that my special skill, my deeper insight, and my "walking in their shoes" helped them through a calmer life and into a better world.

My clients and their friends and relatives have given me a wealth of knowledge that I use as I stumble along, grasping for more. They've whetted my curiosity about themselves and their private worlds, and often they've assuaged that curiosity. I may be a bit crazier for all that I've experienced (the blow to the head didn't help), but I hope I am also wiser. And I hope when the time comes for me to face my own aging, frailty, illness, disability, and/or loneliness, there will be someone to hold me up, push me along, and walk a mile or two in my shoes.

Preface

Home healthcare is this country's fastest growing industry. The sixty-five-and-older population is projected to increase to 15 percent (more than thirty-nine million) by 2010. According to the National Alliance for Caregiving, 22 million families (nearly one in four) already provide assistance to an older relative or friend.

To the vast number of people growing older, add those who are younger, but disabled or ill, and the need for homecare looms even more formidable. As baby boomers age into their fifties, sixties, and seventies over the next thirty years, the need for homecare may prove unmanageable with the resources currently available. The numbers associated with homecare are daunting and the search for a homeworker may seem futile.

But take heart. However difficult finding an accomplished, caring homeworker may be or however stressful taking a stranger into your home may seem, it can be done.

The purpose of this book is to make the homecare process, whether long- or short-term, easier for clients, advocates, and caregivers. The following pages are filled with practical information, tools with which to build efficient and effective homecare settings.

When I began writing two years ago, tired and frustrated from having worked in home healthcare for many years, I used that fatigue and frustration as motivation to keep writing. Knowing certain answers to difficult questions about homecare, I felt it important to share that information with others.

In converting the information to text, I encountered several style problems and solved them in these ways:

I have used singular case pronouns in most cases, as we will be talking about situations that usually are one on one. Fighting differentiation of the sexes, because we're all in this together, I have used nouns instead of pronouns, wherever possible. Client is used, instead of elder, patient, or loved one, because there are no age or familial parameters within homecare. Not everyone needing assistance is ill, and not all care recipients will be one of the reader's loved ones. Client also implies respect within a business arrangement, which homecare is. I protected the privacy of past clients by making each personal anecdote a composite of several characters representative of a particular homecare situation.

Homecare, The Best is divided into three sections. Each section is dedicated to either the client, the advocate, or the homeworker. These are the three main participants in the homecare process. Each participant is advised to read not only their own section, but also the sections addressed to the other two participants. If each participant acquires understanding of the special perspectives of the other two, the homecare process will be less confusing, less exhausting, and less stressful.

Section I shows clients how to choose advocates and how to locate, pay for, and live with homeworkers.

Section II gives advocates valuable information and sensible tips about giving a client (a friend or family member) support.

Section III is for caregivers and domestic workers. (Throughout the book *both* kinds of workers are referred to as homeworkers.) From reading this section, all homeworkers can gain further knowledge about the crucial roles they assumed when they entered the field of healthcare or domestic service.

The appendices contain titles for further reading and the names and numbers of organizations from which all three homecare participants can receive valuable information and support.

And speaking of support, I want to acknowledge and thank those who have supported me in the writing of this book: dear friends, Patty Lou Bryan, Carol Strite, and Mickey Strickland; wise co-workers, Josie Walker, Katie Howard-Melchor, Barbara Lewicki, and Steve Stevens; and ever-faithful family members, Mayfred "Granny" Whatley, Sonja, Sarina, Misty Leigh, Sam, Patricia, and my deceased father, Edward, who still watches. For Walter, thanks will never be enough.

My gratitude and appreciation go to Ellen Lambert, Elizabeth Simmons, and Jihan Rohbacker for their professional opinions and invaluable suggestions.

Humor has always been a saving grace for me, but with the seriousness of the subject at hand, I felt levity to be out of place in this text. However, it was laughter (sometimes laughter mixed with tears) that kept my clients, their families, and me from giving up completely.

I want to wish every client success in this adventure, because this alteration in life, welcome or not, is indeed that: an adventure. And for the client's friends, relatives, and advocates, I wish clear direction and wisdom. And for the caregiver or homeworker who knows much, but who can always learn more, I wish compassion, empathy, and patience, patience, patience.

SECTION I

The Client: The Care Recipient

No wise man [or woman] ever wished to be younger.
Jonathan Swift

1

The Homecare Process

Personal assistance, medical care, companionship—you need one, perhaps all. The reason is age, illness, or disability and you, the client, have determined that you need or will need part-time or full-time help.

Before reaching for this book you may have considered other care options such as group homes, nursing homes, retirement communities, assisted living facilities, and homes of relatives. However, your main desire is to stay at home and have help come to you. You have decided upon or are considering homecare.

Bessie, age 79

I've had a live-in health aide for three months now, and I'm just getting used to having her here.

I tried living with my daughter, Leslie, because I kept falling, but at my age, three teenagers and a four-year-old can break your last nerve.

So I moved in with my son, Jed, but his wife got on my nerves worse. Everything had a place and where I put something wasn't it. She thought I should go to a "home." Well, I knew I had *some* say.

That's when I decided to use my savings to take care of me instead of worrying about leaving it all behind. It was surely worth the money to stay in my own place with my own things. On weekends my kids and grand-kids look in on me, and I'm real careful of myself.

When you begin your search for a homeworker, you are facing a six-step process:

1. Choosing an **advocate**.
2. Deciding the **type** of care you need.
3. Finding a **source** for that type of care.
4. Determining the **cost** of that care and to **pay** for it.
5. Choosing a homeworker, by **interviewing** and **verifying** information, who is compatible with you.
6. **Learning to live with that worker in your home**.

Now is the time to take stock and make note of your potential support network: family members, friends, neighbors, doctors, senior support groups, reference publications, and this book. Take advantage of the knowledge and insight you glean from these sources. By doing so, you will smooth out the rough spots you are sure to encounter in your search for the homeworker most suited to your needs.

2

Choosing an Advocate

Even the hardiest soul will want and need an advocate, someone to stand up and speak out when hard questions or difficult situations arise. This person will assist you in making phone calls, filling out paperwork, conducting interviews, and attending to the countless details involved in the homecare process. At times, with your permission, your advocate may serve as your surrogate when there are choices or decisions to be made.

When you choose an advocate, keep in mind that energy, patience, persistence, and curiosity are the most desirable traits for a person serving in that capacity. If you have a problem to solve and your advocate isn't up for the challenge, the problem may become an even larger problem.

Inez, age 60

I've always had a problem asserting myself and doing any kind of business. I guess I'm one of those people who is naturally shy.

When I realized I needed someone to stay with me after my stroke, I was scared. But Elle, the pastor's wife, had always been real sweet and had told me if I ever needed anything, to let her know.

I hated to ask for help, Elle was always so busy. But she stepped in and was just wonderful.

After a couple of months, I was settled at home with all the help I needed, and Elle assured me she was just a call away. Somehow, having someone with her energy and self assurance in my corner makes me feel protected, safe.

Your advocate might feel close enough to you—be interested enough in you as a friend or family member—that money will be of no consideration. If you feel that money will be an issue . . .

DISCUSS—DECIDE—PUT IT IN WRITING!

You will see the above phrase or variations of it throughout this book. The phrase is set in caps and typed in boldface for good reason: to get your attention and urge you to act now so you can avoid headaches and heartaches later.

Please, if you ignore any advice contained within the pages that follow, do not let it be this important directive. Between you and the people who work for you, little misunderstandings can lead to big complications. Having a written agreement can save everyone involved a lot of grief.

3

Finding the Type of Caregiver/ Homeworker You Need

Below are listed the five main types of homeworkers and a comprehensive description of the duties performed by each.

Homemaker

A homemaker performs household chores that include some or all of the following:

- Meal planning and preparation
- Shopping assistance
- Sweeping, mopping, vacuuming, and waxing floors
- Dusting and washing woodwork, cleaning *inside* windows, dusting and polishing furniture (and valuable collectibles you care to trust to another's hands)
- Cleaning bathroom fixtures and surfaces
- Laundering and ironing household linens
- Cleaning kitchen surfaces and appliances

The following duties are optional and should be discussed independently and agreed upon between the client and the homemaker:

- Laundering and ironing personal clothing

- Errand running
- Driving to medical appointments
- Pet care
- Valet services
- Plant care and outside chores
- Mail retrieval if mail is picked up at a mail box center or post office

If your home is small, a housekeeper may agree to assume additional duties—at no additional cost to you. You will have to . . .

DISCUSS—DECIDE—PUT IT IN WRITING.

To put it in writing, simply type or write out the following form, and then fill it out.

Resolution Form   Date_____

An agreement between: _____

and   _____

Pertaining to:_____

_____

It is agreed that:_____

_____

_____

Signed_____Date:_____
                        Client
Signed_____ Date:_____
                     Homeworker

Keep a file of signed Resolution Forms for all home-workers and make sure homeworkers receive a copy of each form they sign.

Companion

A large number of aging, ill, lonely, or disabled clients find a companion a great asset. Besides people who work independently as companions, there are agencies (either "sitter" agencies or homemaker/sitter/companion agencies) that specialize in placing this type of worker in private homes. In some states these agencies must be licensed and/or registered with the state, and they must screen workers before placing them with clients.

For a companion or sitter there is no rigid job description, but it is generally accepted that a person working in this capacity will:

- Help the client with correspondence and assist with telephone business such as setting appointments
- Accompany client on social, family, or business outings, when asked
- Drive, run errands, and attend to mail
- Help with pet and plant care
- Share home entertainment such as games, television, music, and reading

In other words, a companion is an all-around personal assistant, friend, and social aide. You may find a companion who works with a second person, a *tag-team partner,* who fills in when the primary companion worker needs time off. Tag-team partners know each other's work habits and personality, and this preestablished relationship affords you, the client, reliable scheduling and worker compatibility.

Home Health Aide (HHA)

The majority of states require certification for home health aides. Check in your state by calling the telephone number listed in Appendix D. Florida is representative of states with stringent qualification guidelines for home health aides. They require at least forty hours, and sometimes as much as seventy-five hours, of training and the passing of a state test.

In states that issue HHA certificates, the aide must keep a daily diary of activities performed with and by the client. An HHA must also list medications taken by the client and the time those medications were taken. It is important to note that an aide cannot directly administer medication. An aide can only *offer* a pill bottle or pill organizer (a compartmentalized container) to the client, so the client can select the medication. Generally, a home health aide performs the following duties:

- Assists client in movement into and out of bed, wheelchair, or automobile, up and down stairs, and to and from the bathroom
- Assists client with personal grooming, bathing, and dressing
- Changes the bed linens, attends to client's personal laundry, and keeps client's surroundings clean and neat
- Prepares and serves food for the client and self only, and prepares special diets as directed by the client or the client's physician
- Participates in client's daily activities (playing games, watching TV, reading aloud, listening to music, watching movies)
- Food shopping by the HHA may or may not be required, and, if it is, providing a car for trips to the supermarket is primarily the client's responsibility

(In some instances, HHAs hired through an agency are not allowed to drive a client's car for *any* reason.)

If you allow a worker to drive your car, consult your insurance agent about liability and responsibility for that worker as a driver.

Regarding the worker's use of your car and possibly cooking for your spouse . . .

DISCUSS—DECIDE—PUT IT IN WRITING!

Virginia, age 57

My husband, Steve, had reached the final stage of emphysema. I had my hands full with our home, our business, and his ongoing care. I finally had to admit I needed help and called a healthcare agency through which I hired two homeworkers: a home health aide and a nurse assistant. I thought I had all bases covered.

The very first meal prepared by the home health aide was for herself and my husband. There was no plate set for me. The aide explained that she could look after and cook for Steve, but none of her services were to overlap to me. "Agency rules," she said.

After talking with the agency supervisor who verified what the aide had told me, I began a search of my own. By asking around, talking to people I knew at my club and at church, I hired two women, one was a homemaker and the other would cook for both my husband and myself. For Steve's personal needs, I had the agency send in a nurse assistant four times a week.

I wish the agency had been more clear, as a better understanding on my part would have saved me a lot of precious time and energy.

A word of caution: Before hiring a home health aide instead of another type of homeworker, check state regulations. If you require any kind of medical assistance, you may need a worker who is licensed to deliver services that an HHA is not licensed to deliver.

Nurse Aide (NA)/Certified Nurse Aide (CNA)

Regulations and licensing requirements for a nurse aide (also called nurse assistant or nursing assistant) vary from state to state, and some states may require certification for those aides who work in private homes as well as for those who work in institutional settings. An aide becomes certified by completing a state required course and then passing a state administered test. Again, representative of more stringent state requirements are those of Florida. Nurse aide certification in that state requires 120 to 300 hours of training, the passing of a state test, continuing education credits, and periodic renewal of certification. If a nurse aide also wants to work as an HHA, another twenty hours of training is mandatory.

Home healthcare agencies (which we will discuss in detail shortly) require proof of certification from an aide before placing that aide in a private home and you should, too. Certification verifies that the nurse aide has had state required training and is adept in transport and movement of clients, range of motion, the taking of vital signs, manipulation of physical aids and restraints, measurement of intake and output, and the collection of specimens, as well as personal care skills. When working under the supervision of a licensed nurse (a registered nurse or a licensed practical nurse) a nurse aide can perform other, more complex services.

Even if certification of a nurse aide for homecare is not mandatory in your state, it is a plus for you and your future care, because in many states a nurse aide *does* need certification to provide the client with in-hospital care. If you spend time in the hospital, you may be denied the added comfort of care from the nurse aide who has provided your in-home care. Keep this in mind as you assess your present and possible future needs.

Licensed Practical Nurse(LPN)/Registered Nurse (R.N.)

For this type of worker, licensing is mandatory in all states. Training consists of one year (LPN) and, up to four years (R.N.). A licensed practical nurse or a registered nurse can administer medications in either oral doses or by injection.

Other duties allowed by R.N.s and LPNs but not allowed by HHAs and CNAs are administering intravenous therapy, drawing blood (although venipuncture is no longer covered by Medicare), regulating oxygen, changing urinary catheters, instructing in disease management, and reporting effects of medication to a physician.

You now have an idea of the type of homeworker/caregiver you need, so read Step Three for information that will make the search for that homeworker easier.

4

Finding a Source to Provide Your Caregiver/Homeworker

This sounds like an easy undertaking, but finding a good homeworker or caregiver can be a formidable task. One cause for complication in the search is that workers are not cardboard cutouts; they come with varying likes, dislikes, personalities, backgrounds, and experience. Your job is to find the worker most suited to your particular needs, the worker who will become an integral part of your life and help out with activities that you no longer wish to handle alone.

Now is the time for you to compose a complete Need List. Walk through your home, visualize and make notes about everything you need help with or anticipate needing help with.

It is a good idea, if your physical condition permits, to keep some activities and chores for yourself. Continue as usual with activities that present reasonable physical and mental challenges, and also continue those activities that give you a sense of joy or accomplishment. Never use homecare as a crutch, or you will need crutches long before you thought you would. Do be sure that your agreement with a homeworker contains a clause to ensure that the worker will assume those chores should you become unable to perform them. All together, now:

DISCUSS—DECIDE—PUT IT IN WRITING!

Go over your Need List several times, and have your advocate or a friend take an objective final look, then read on to get a clear picture of the different sources of homeworkers, and decide which of those you will use to locate your homeworker.

Source #1: Geriatric care manager

If you, the client, are an older person, you have the option of hiring a professional geriatric care manager to locate, set up, and monitor a network of care. If you are a young person needing homecare, you will call and ask this type of manager if help is available to you.

Care managers work alone or as part of an agency team, and they can serve as valuable adjuncts in planning with your advocate. With their professional expertise and established contacts they can guide you in all phases of setting up and carrying forward a plan of homecare. A care manager may even fill the role of advocate for you. This will be especially helpful if you have no friend or family member to fill that role.

Some care managers specialize in trust, legal, or placement services. Care manager *trust specialists* work with bank trust officers and bank clients and provide assistance with banking and finding homecare or other services tailored to the needs of the trust officer's clients. Care manager *legal specialists* assess and coordinate services for clients under guardianship and for courts and attorneys. The care manager *placement specialist* performs screenings and interviews in-home workers for clients who hire on their own.

All care managers can assist you with:

- Assessing your particular needs and evaluating the level of care you need

- Locating homecare services

- Estimating costs of care

- Keeping medical appointments, making phone calls, running errands

- Investigating and evaluating independent living communities if homecare proves inappropriate for your situation

- Researching and setting up hospice, dementia care, Alzheimer's, and other specialized care, if needed

- Solving the unique problems you may encounter in the homecare situation

Keep in mind that a qualified care manager should have a minimum of a bachelor's degree or verifiable, extensive training in counseling, nursing, gerontology, and/or social work; ask to see diplomas and licenses from any care manger you consult. A good care manager also will have in-depth knowledge about the costs and quality of services in the client's community and the availability of those services.

If you need assistance with locating a qualified care manager in your area, call the National Association of Professional Geriatric Care Managers at the number listed in Appendix C. A care manager will charge $50 to $250 per hour for one or several hours per week. For that fee you should receive caring assistance, valuable information on a wide range of homecare related matters, and practical hands-on homecare management. It is even possible that the care manager can save you a substantial amount of money by using resources that you might never have otherwise found.

Source #2: Friends and Family

The next place to look for a homecare worker is right under your own nose. Ask your physicians, clergyman, neighbors, or club members if they or anyone they know have been through a search for a homeworker. If so, ask if they can recommend a worker to you.

Foregoing the services of a professional care manager, you may find the worker best suited to your needs within your immediate circle of friends and family. Of course, having a friend or family member work for you has both advantages and disadvantages.

The *advantages* are that you already have knowledge about the person. You can skip the search-and-find process, and you avoid paying an agency fee (to certain types of agencies).

The *disadvantages* of having a friend or family worker are that you may find you don't know that person as well as you thought; it is often true that intimacy *does* breed contempt. Also, a friend or family member may lack the skills needed, or be unwilling or lack the patience to perform the services you require. And, lastly, deciding payment for a person close to you can be a delicate issue.

Constance, age 69

After my husband died, I was lonesome and depressed. I thought my niece, Diedre, would be the ideal companion for me. She was young—twenty-eight—but she was a very sweet girl, and had worked for several other elderly ladies.

Alas, dear me. After two weeks, I knew I had made a mistake. For one thing, Diedre gossiped about everyone. She was constantly on the phone and she had personal errands to run every single day.

I discreetly called one of her past employers who said Diedre had done none of these things while employed by her. I concluded that working for her own aunt just didn't seem like a real job to Diedre.

She was understanding when I voiced my concerns, and she kept coming over until I found a companion through a placement agency.

I regret having put my niece and myself in such an awkward situation. Even now when I see Diedre, I still feel a little guilty about it all.

As you can see, establishing a homeworker relationship with a friend or family member can be fraught with problems, and such an arrangement should be avoided, unless you know that the person you are considering is naturally giving and patient in other types of relationships.

If you have the slightest doubt about an arrangement of this sort, cross it off your list. Do not risk losing a valued friend or family member by attempting to establish a new and difficult relationship. In the future, you might find that the very person you considered as a caregiver will become, instead, your strongest advocate.

Harold, age 91

I asked my daughter, Mary Margaret, what good was she if she couldn't look after me. Her mother always took care of everything.

After my wife passed, someone had to keep things going . . . my accounts as well as the house. What the hell did I know about it. I've run my own business all my life, never had time for anything else.

Mary Margaret could have done it all, but she wouldn't . . . said she couldn't. Kept losing her temper with me, crying, carrying on.

Then, without asking me, she called her brother. My son, Malcolm, is a CEO, runs his own consulting firm. He knew what to do. He had his sec-

> retary find me a cook, a homemaker, and a driver all in one. He found a CPA to come by every week, too. Smart boy.
>
> Mary Margaret calls, runs some errands for me. Guess I can thank her for that little bit, but I'll just never understand that girl.

If you are fortunate enough to find a suitable caregiver/domestic worker in your immediate circle of contacts, be sure you give that person the same respect and consideration that you would give a professionally trained homecare worker. And, impersonal as it may seem, be professional in this way: Have a long, sincere talk with that friend or family member and . . .

DISCUSS—DECIDE—PUT EVERYTHING IN WRITING.

Source #3: Newspaper Classifieds

You can search for a homeworker in your newspaper; qualified workers (and sometimes *un*qualified workers—beware) often list in newspaper classified ads.

The *one real advantage* of hiring from a classified ad is that you have no middleman to pay; you will not pay a domestic agency's or a homemaker/sitter/companion agency's fee or a nurse registry fee. (A fourth type of agency, the home healthcare agency, usually does not charge a fee to place a worker.)

The *disadvantages* are several. You and/or your advocate will have no one to carry out background checks or conduct preliminary interviews, you will have no agency buffer or feedback, and you and/or your advocate will spend time and energy answering or placing ads and arranging interviews. Without doubt, you will feel more secure and be less harried if you use a source other than newspaper classifieds to find the worker you need.

If you decide you want to use classified ads, have an advocate by your side to help you interview and screen applicants and to assist you in making a final hiring decision. A second set of perceptions and opinions when hiring from this source is absolutely necessary.

Source #4: Volunteer or Government Agencies

Other non-agency sources to contact are groups affiliated with your church, volunteer organizations, and local, state, or national agencies. Two of the latter are the Area Agencies on Aging (AAA) and Children of Aging Parents (CAPS). Both are excellent sources of information and referrals. (Contact numbers for these and other support organizations are listed in Appendix C, and state Area Agencies on Aging are listed in Appendix E.)

Source #5 Medicare

The information given here about Medicare is current at this time, but you should check all guidelines before using them for planning homecare.

The last wide-reaching changes to Medicare homecare coverage were instituted with the passing of the Balanced Budget Act of 1997. The most significant change at that time erased the differences in homecare coverage connected to a hospital stay as opposed to homecare coverage provided *without* a hospital stay. Coverage guidelines are now the same for both situations. For the most up-to-date information on Medicare homecare coverage, you will call the Social Security Administration, Medicare, a nurse registry, or a home healthcare agency in your community.

Medicare does not cover long-term homecare, but if you, the client, are eligible for Medicare, you may qualify for injury or illness related short-term/rehabilitative homecare that can last up to six months. Medicare homecare benefits cannot be accessed for conditions related solely to aging or nonmedical frailty. Injury or illness related home healthcare services are available under either Part A or Part B of Medicare.

Medicare Part A is hospitalization insurance that is automatically included in Social Security benefits. Medicare Part B is optional medical insurance, which is paid with a monthly premium that can be deducted from the client's monthly Social Security payment. Check to see if you qualify for Medicare under any of the following conditions. If you do not, you may still be able to buy in and enroll in Medicare *if you are sixty-five or older.*

To be *eligible* automatically for Medicare you must:
1. Be age sixty-five or older and have worked long enough and paid in an adequate amount to be insured under federal employment, the railroad retirement system, or Social Security *or:*
2. Already be receiving railroad retirement or Social Security benefits *or:*
3. Be entitled to Medicare because you have permanent kidney failure *or:*
4. Be under sixty-five, disabled per Medicare definition and decision, and have been entitled to Social Security for the twenty-four months previous to your need for homecare.

Then, to be *qualified* for the short-term, rehabilitative services you need, all four of the following conditions must be met:

1. A physician must determine that you need home healthcare, set up a plan of care for you, and continue supervision of that plan with you under his or her care.
2. You must need certain types of care as outlined by Medicare, and this care must include part-time

skilled nursing care, physical therapy or speech therapy. After you no longer need these types of care, Medicare can still pay for prescribed home healthcare visits if you need *occupational* therapy.

3. You must be confined to your home—*homebound*. The Medicare definition of homebound does not require that you, the client, be bedridden, but you must have a normal *inability* to leave the home without *considerable* and *taxing* effort.

4. The home healthcare agency that provides the homecare workers that you need is approved by and actively participating in the Medicare program.

For the client to receive the *non-skilled services* of a home health aide, the client must qualify for skilled home health care under Medicare guidelines, the HHA services must be part-time or intermittent, and the services must be reasonable and necessary to the treatment of the client's diagnosed medical condition. Further:

• The HHA must provide hands-on personal care that is needed to maintain the client's health or facilitate treatment of the client's illness or injury.

• The frequency of HHA visits must be indicated by a physician.

• Services must be those allowed by an HHA, and may include bathing, dressing, caring for hair, nail, and oral hygiene needed to facilitate treatment or prevent deterioration of the client's health; changing bed linens for an incontinent client; shaving, deodorant application, skin care with lotions and/or powder; foot care, and ear care. Depending on state guidelines, services of an HHA may also include feeding, assistance with elimination (including enemas unless skilled care is needed because of the client's condition), routine catheter care, routine colostomy care, assistance with walking, patient positioning in bed, and assistance with transfers.

Home healthcare services completely *excluded* by Medicare are long-term homecare, medicines, blood transfusions, personal comfort items, full-time nursing care, venipuncture, homemaker services, and meals delivered to your home.

William, age 40

I had always thought Medicare took care of old people, no matter who they were or what the problem was. Two years ago I found out I was wrong.

I lived in Florida; my mother lived in New York. It took me three visits and hundreds of phone calls before I accepted the fact that she was "losing it." She was finally diagnosed with senile dementia.

All my aunts and uncles were elderly. I was her only child, and in poor health. With only Social Security and a small pension, she couldn't afford the care—custodial, not medical—that she needed.

My friends said Medicare would pay for help, so I talked to the people at the Medicare office. I learned that Medicare would pay only for recuperation and rehabilitation from an injury or illness. My mother would have to have a health problem that could be cured or improved, but all she really needed was a friendly bodyguard.

The answer for her was Medicaid. It took two months to get through the red tape and get homecare, but now she's safe from leaving pot holders on lit burners and wandering the neighborhood at all hours.

You can receive a publication that explains Medicare's homecare coverage by calling the number listed for the Social Security Administration in Appendix C. Easier for you to understand will be one of the additional recommended readings listed in Appendix B. At your local library the reference librarian can locate for you numerous publications that contain detailed information on Medicare.

Source #6: Medicaid

Medicaid is a state/federal program that provides medical and medically related assistance to aged, blind, and disabled low-income individuals, as well as to medically needy families with children. *Medically needy* means that household income is considered insufficient to cover both living expenses and medical care within the household. To locate the Medicaid office in your area look in the telephone book under federal government listings such as "Health Care Administration Agency."

Unlike Medicare, Medicaid (Medi-Cal in California) *does* cover some long-term homecare and other services such as homemaker services and meals delivered to your home.

Eligibility for Medicaid is based on the following factors, and dollar amounts vary from state to state.

1. If you are eligible for Medicare, benefits under Medicare must be used before Medicaid benefits become accessible.

2. You must meet *maximum* income limits (you cannot receive income over a certain amount). Income includes all regular, recurring payments to you such as wages, unemployment insurance, Social Security income, pensions, dividends, interest, cash contributions from friends and family, and business profits. Remember, maximum income limits vary from state to state.

3. Your assets must include nothing more than (a) a car, (b) personal and household items, (c) a burial plot and

Homemaker / Sitter / Companion Agency. In most states there are two types of homemaker/sitter/companion agencies (referred to as h/s/c agencies from here on): (1) Those that are state registered and authorized to place a homemaker, sitter, or companion with an elderly, handicapped, or convalescent person, and (2) those that are not.

If the h/s/c agency is state registered, it can place workers who will accompany clients on trips and outings, prepare and serve meals, and stabilize the client during walking, standing, or sitting. Those workers, however, cannot provide personal health care services that an HHA or a CNA can provide. Your need for assistance must be minimal if you are to use this type of agency.

A state registered h/s/c agency is required to do the following:

- Verify workers' employment histories and refuse agency listing to any worker who will not provide information for verification
- Inform the client of the right to report abusive, neglectful, or exploitative practices by the worker
- Display its registration number in all advertising
- Have minimum standards ensuring that no worker has been found guilty or pleaded guilty to any of a number of criminal charges as listed by the state
- Keep current and hold registration that shows it has filed information under oath about the person or persons (owner or owners of the agency) who provide workers for its listed services

If the h/s/c agency is not state registered and holds only a business license, it cannot legally place workers with elderly, handicapped, or convalescent clients who may need more than ordinary companionship and assistance. If you, the client, require any kind of personal care or medical assistance, this agency will be unable to fill your needs.

Nurse Registry. A nurse registry is run by one or more persons who place R.N.s, LPNs, CNAs, HHAs, and perhaps homemakers, sitters, and companions as independent contractors (discussion and description of independent contractors, page 55). This type of agency places workers in private homes and institutional settings, and in all states operating requirements are much the same.

Important points for the client to know about a nurse registry are the following:

- A registry must be licensed as a nurse registry and operate within state and federal guidelines.

- A registry enters into a contract with the client and serves only to procure, offer, promise, or attempt to secure healthcare for the client.

- A registry makes sure that workers meet state independent contractor registration requirements.

- A registry provides no payroll services, because the worker's relationship with the agency is that of independent contractor.

- A registry must make sure that a client is under a physician's care before placing a CNA or any provider of medical assistance in the client's home.

- A registry must have an R.N. make visits to the client's home as proscribed by state regulations to assess the client's condition and the quality of care being provided by the CNA.

- A registry requires that every worker complete an agency application form that contains certain personal history, education and employment history, and the number and date of the worker's professional license. Using this information, the agency must screen the worker and maintain an information file on that worker.

Before beginning the hiring process through a nurse registry, be sure that you fully understand the services the registry can provide. If you prefer interacting directly with a homeworker and do not mind setting up a payroll system or have someone handle payroll for you, then you may want to hire through this type of agency. However, you may prefer having another party serve as the direct employer and serve as a buffer between you and a worker, and the services of a home healthcare agency may be more to your liking.

Home Healthcare Agency. A home healthcare agency is an agency whose business consists of developing care plans, placing healthcare workers in private homes and institutions, and supervising the workers it places.

Representative of one of the most common types of home healthcare agency is the Visiting Nurse Association (VNA) with offices nationwide providing healthcare and custodial workers such as R.N.s, LPNs, HHAs, medical social workers, homemakers, companions, and physical, occupational, and speech therapists. Each VNA is operated locally and run by a volunteer board of directors; there is no "home" office and no private owner(s). (A national number for referral to VNA offices is listed in Appendix C.)

VNA operates as a *not-for-profit* healthcare agency and usually does not ask for a deposit before services begin. This type of agency pays a worker directly and is reimbursed by Medicare, Medicaid, private insurance, or the client. The agency administers a payroll accounting plan and makes mandatory deductions and withholdings from payments to workers.

This type of agency is rigidly monitored by state and federal authorities. Following is a *partial and simplified* list of standards under which it operates.

- Licenses must be renewed annually, and financial ability to provide services must be documented.
- Owners and/or directors must pass an FBI background check.
- City and county occupational licenses must be renewed each year, and proof of bonding of agency employees providing services must be submitted.
- Employees of the agency are required to undergo physicals, test for TB, receive Hepatitis B shots, and undergo drug screening.
- Employee licenses and training must be validated by the agency and an orientation program maintained for all new employees.
- The agency must keep Workers' Compensation coverage for employees and withhold federal taxes from employee wages.

Client services provided by VNA and home health-care agencies of a similar nature are many. An agency in compliance with state and federal government standards will, at least, do the following:

- Establish policies drawn up by a professional group associated with the agency. The professional group will include at least one physician and one registered nurse.
- Make diligent effort to verify worker information and screen each worker. Screening includes an employment history check, a check of references, a check of the state abuse registry, and a criminal history check.
- Verify that all workers have state and federal required training, certificates, and licenses.
- Take responsibility for all services delivered to clients by agency personnel.
- Accept clients who need skilled services and also those who need the non-skilled services of a home-maker, sitter, or companion.

- Draw up and follow a care plan for each client to whom services are delivered.
- Keep a detailed clinical record and a confidential file of each client.
- Have an R.N. supervise services that are delivered by an LPN or an HHA.
- Evaluate the appropriateness of homemaker services every six months.
- Act as direct employer to its workers and assume payroll accounting duties.
- File medical claims for clients.
- Make sure that workers are bonded and insured.
- Mediate homecare related problems between the worker and the client.

When shopping for a home healthcare agency, refer to the list above and ask questions on each point. Agency personnel will know that you are looking for the best of homecare and that you, the client, and your advocate have more than a passing concern about the services the agency can provide. Many hospitals are affiliated with a homecare agency that operates under a hospital associated name: Parrish Medical Center—Parrish HomeCare. When you are discharged from a hospital, the hospital social services representative can assist you with setting up a plan of homecare, but you are by no means obligated to use the affiliated agency, which may be either a for-profit or a not-for-profit business.

Unlike a not-for-profit agency, a *for-profit* healthcare agency will often charge an up-front fee (similar to a placement fee charged by a domestic staffing agency). A for-profit healthcare agency must be licensed to place healthcare workers, normally does not receive reimbursement from Medicare or Medicaid (the client or insurance company will pay for services), and determines for itself the margin of profit at which it will operate. The client may be required to pay a deposit before services begin and is billed weekly or monthly for continuing services. Out of the amounts remitted by the client or insurance company, the agency computes payroll amounts and deductions and then pays a worker a set hourly, weekly, or per-visit amount.

Bev, age 67

There's never been a problem I couldn't solve, a challenge I couldn't meet. And I *always* did my research. So, when I decided to hire a person to help with my housework and errands, I got out the phone book and went to work.

I found a woman through a staffing agency, paid their fee (a hefty $2,000), then spent several intense weeks showing her the ropes and getting acquainted.

Then my car broke down and I asked my helper to use her car to run my errands. She said, "Sorry, no way." I called the agency to see what the policy about car use was.

Mrs. Porey, the director, said that once the helper had been placed with me, the agency had no further responsibility in the relationship. She did offer to speak to the helper in my behalf. I said, "Thank you, but I'll do it myself."

My helper and I discussed the issue, and I agreed to pay her gas and $15 to cover wear and tear on her car.

My experience enlightened me about the different kinds of agencies. Some take care of settling things like that, and some of them just don't.

As you can see, there is much to consider. Take your time, assume nothing, and exercise deliberate care and consideration before choosing an agency.

Before you leave this chapter on the sources of help, look at two additional sources that provide homeworkers in special circumstances: hospice and managed care.

Source #6: Hospice

To receive *hospice* care, a client must have a life-limiting (terminal) illness and be unable to benefit from ongoing curative treatment(s). Services available from hospice include pain and symptom control, counseling, spiritual care, respite care for family and caregivers, and coordination of care.

To be admitted to hospice and receive homecare services, a client must sign a "hospice election form," which states that the client understands that the treatment involved is aimed at pain relief and symptom control and not curative treatment. If covered by Medicare, the client must understand how entering hospice affects Medicare coverage for a terminal illness. The most difficult part of signing these forms and entering hospice is that the client has to acknowledge that life expectancy at that point is no more than six months. This is a requirement of receiving the valuable and comforting homecare services that hospice can provide.

If you qualify for hospice and want to stay in your own home, homecare services will be available to you. These include the services of a physician, nurses, and other professionals working in tandem with a primary caregiver who is most often the spouse or a member of the client's immediate family. In the privacy of a home setting, the client can receive nursing care, pharmacy services, and physician services around the clock.

Hospice is funded by a variety of sources that include Medicare, Medicaid (in some states), the Veterans Administration, some private insurance plans, private payment, health maintenance organizations, and other managed care programs. If a client has inadequate or no financial resources to pay for hospice, most hospices provide services free of charge. (Refer to Appendix C for a contact number and Appendix B for an Internet address.)

Source #7: Managed Care

The words *managed care* may bring to mind for a client an arrangement for delivery of healthcare services called a health maintenance organization (HMO). More attractive to that client might be a similar organization like the Program of All-Inclusive Care for the Elderly, which currently operates in only certain states. PACE, however, is not a private for-profit health maintenance organization, but a program that is sanctioned, funded and monitored by state and federal governments. As such, the program operates under strict regulations.

PACE targets long-term care for clients fifty-five and older. In Colorado, the program is administered by Total Longterm Care, which oversees several sites in the Denver area. The program allows a client to remain at home and still receive an array of medical, social, and custodial services. If nursing home care should become necessary, PACE manages that care as well.

Available services include primary care, social work, and restorative therapy. Also, specialty and ancillary medical services are provided, as are long-term care services such as transportation, meals, and personal care. PACE provides speech therapy, nutrition counseling, chore services, escort service, and recreation therapy. These services are paid for with Medicare and Medicaid capitation payments (payment made for each person served) and private payments from clients ineligible for

Medicare and Medicaid. (To inquire about PACE administration and center locations in your state call the number listed in Appendix C.)

With your advocate and your Need List at hand, proceed to Step Four, Determining Cost and Paying for Care. With the knowledge you now have about different types of agencies and the information contained in this next step, you will be able to define a clear homecare plan.

5

Determining Costs and Paying for Care

To cut the costs of homecare, consider coordinating care by using different types and sources of caregivers. You may want a home-health aide or a nurse aide to come to your home for only an hour or two each day to give assistance with personal care, then enlist a friend to run errands for you.

If coordinating care and cutting costs in this manner is not an option, you will pay for a homeworker's services as outlined under the following headings.

Cost/Payment #1: Friends or Family

Explore the possibilities of friends, family members, and neighbors piecing together the services you need. If successful in finding care within your circle of friends and family, you will be free to determine payment and perks among yourselves. If in doubt about a fair rate of pay, consult the chart, page 59. Who knows? For you, those friends and family members may be able to volunteer their services. However, do not assume that friends or family members—with or without fair compensation— will be able to assist you.

Cost/Payment #2: Newspaper Classified Ads

Finding a homeworker through newspaper classified ads (either placing an ad or answering one) will eliminate your paying an up-front fee to a nurse registry, domestic staffing agency, an h/s/c agency or a for-profit healthcare agency. That worker will, however, usually expect a pay rate equal to that of an agency-based worker. (See chart, page 59.) If a worker you hire through an ad is willing to accept a very low rate of pay, be wary. Although the worker may have legitimate reasons for accepting lower pay, be sure you know what those reasons are.

Cost/Payment #3: Volunteer Organizations

Often, charity or church sponsored agencies provide homeworkers who accept payment on a sliding scale for clients unable to pay full hourly, weekly, or shift rates. Some even have qualified workers who volunteer their skills. There are a number of national support, information, and referral organizations that can steer you to sources of help and charge you little or nothing for their assistance. (See Appendix C for telephone numbers.)

Cost/Payment #4: Medicare

Medicare does not pay for custodial care or care needed because of frailty. Care must be deemed medically necessary, and it must serve to rehabilitate the client.

Under Part A, Medicare pays 100 percent of services for care delivered under Medicare guidelines and standards—the client pays nothing. Medicare also pays 80 percent of the approved amount on durable medical equipment (wheelchairs, canes, hospital beds, etc.), and the client pays the remaining 20 percent. Under Part B, Medicare pays the same amounts for medical care and durable equipment as under Part A.

Cost/Payment #5: Medicaid

For those clients who qualify, Medicaid may pay some overflow costs from Medicare. Medicaid also may cover some custodial care at no charge to the client.

Cost/Payment #6: Agencies

Domestic staffing agencies collect from the client an up-front or placement fee usually equal to four to six times the worker's weekly wage. If the client is going to pay the worker $400 per week, the placement fee could be $2,400.

For the placement fee charged, the agency guarantees the client's satisfaction with the worker, but only for a limited time, usually four to eight weeks. If for any reason during that period the client/worker relationship becomes untenable, the agency provides a replacement worker and charges *no additional fee*.

If you hire a worker through a domestic staffing agency (or a classified ad, or some types of h/s/c and healthcare agencies), you are responsible for payroll arrangements, so be clear about the worker's status under Internal Revenue Service guidelines.

Under IRS guidelines, a person who is *self-employed* usually owns a licensed business and provides services or goods directly to a wholesale or retail consumer. The self-employed person has a named business and advertises under that name. The IRS requires that self-employed persons pay self-employment tax, which includes Social Security, Medicare, and income tax payments.

A person who works independently for you usually will not meet the IRS conditions set forth for a self-employed person. The person working independently (not under a business name and not as an employee of an agency) is considered by the IRS to be either an *independent contractor* or *your direct employee*.

For you, the client, to avoid trouble with the IRS, be sure that a worker claiming independent contractor status works for you under these conditions and

- pays all federal, state, and local taxes on income;
- pays all Social Security and Medicare (FICA) taxes;
- reports fees of $600 or more that you pay in wages on Form 1099-MISC;
- sets out and controls the hours to be worked;
- decides which services to provide to you, and
- provides all equipment necessary to perform services.

If a worker provides services under these conditions, it means that the *worker* retains control over how and when services will be delivered, and that the client has a say about only the end result of his or her efforts. In homecare this is not the usual working relationship.

Most often, a homeworker hired through a classified ad, a domestic staffing agency, a nurse registry, or an h/s/c agency and paid directly by you, the client, works as an *employee*. If you hire a worker through a not-for-profit home healthcare agency, that worker will still be an employee, but not your direct employee. That worker will be an employee of the agency who is providing services to you. An employee who works *directly for you*

- follows a job schedule set by you, the client, (arrives and leaves at times set by you);
- renders services requested by you and provides those services in compliance with your instructions, and
- uses equipment provided by you to perform job duties.

As a direct employer for any worker that you pay $1,000 or more per year, you, the client, have responsibilities under IRS guidelines which include

- Having each new worker fill out a W-4 form, the

withholding allowance certificate that shows identifying information and exemptions for a worker

- Withholding required income tax amounts from wages—optional, but you want to make sure that the worker is filing yearly estimated tax payments and that you will not be held liable for tax payments (NOTE: The client can pay income taxes for a worker, but must count that payment as additional wages to the worker. This additional amount is not considered wages for Social Security and Medicare tax purposes.)

- Paying half of Social Security and Medicare payments and making sure that the worker is paying the other half

  If you do not withhold the worker's share of these payments, you can be liable for the full amount.

- Paying state required amounts for Workers Compensation (Mandatory if the client employs a certain number of workers.)

- Paying required amounts for federal unemployment taxes

  Bottom line: A client pays out more for an employee than for an independent contractor, but the client is sure that all payments required by the IRS are paid.

If your worker insists upon working as self-employed or as an independent contractor, be sure to have that worker complete and sign the Internal Revenue form W-9, (taxpayer identification number and certification form). Keep an original signed copy for yourself. The signed form is a worker's official declaration that you have been given a correct tax identification number (usually a Social Security number). This form ensures you against having to pay "backup" withholding and/or taxes that a worker claiming independent contractor status should have paid. (See Appendix B for further reading and Appendix C for the IRS telephone number.)

DO NOT DISCUSS—JUST DO IT!

Evelyn, age 68

Charleen came to me through a church referral in January, 1996. I was happy to find someone who I assumed had been checked out by the church.

When Charleen started, she wanted her weekly pay intact and said she would take care of her taxes and everything. That took a load off me, as I knew nothing about those things.

Well, Charleen slept so soundly and snored so loudly that she kept me awake. She couldn't even hear my monitor beeper when I needed her. So we talked, and she left the last of May 1996.

In late March 1997, Mr. Wormar, my banker, called to tell me that Charleen wanted me to pay her Social Security and Medicare. She said I was *supposed* to. After talking to Mr. Wormar and making several calls to the IRS, this is what I learned:

Charleen had worked as an employee, and if I wasn't going to withhold from her check, I should have had her sign a TIN Form, and for my own protection, have her declare in writing that she was working as an independent contractor.

To settle things, I paid her Social Security and Medicare, and counted myself lucky not to have to pay her taxes. I learned a lesson and, in the future, will make sure to clarify a person's employment status before they come to work for me.

Determine a payroll period, and make sure your homeworker knows before the job begins what that payroll period is. Most workers prefer to be paid weekly, and indeed, writing smaller checks more often may be less painful for you, the client. If you have a banker or an accountant who provides payroll service, give that professional the worker's rate of pay and leave the figuring to them.

There are also payroll service companies that provide the same services that bankers or accountants provide. For under $50 to $100 a month, this type of company will make sure that all proper forms are filed, do all payroll calculations, cut and mail checks, and provide year-end reports for several household employees. You will find these companies listed in the Yellow Pages of your phone book under Payroll Preparation Services.

A nurse registry operates much like a domestic staffing agency, but after collecting a placement fee, a registry does continue to provide minimal services as outlined on page 44.

An h/s/c agency can act as a "placement" agency and charge an up-front fee or it can act as an "employer" agency, and charge the client or insurance company for services and pay the worker a set hourly, daily, weekly, or per-visit rate.

Most for-profit home healthcare agencies collect payment from private-pay clients or private insurance and are paid for worker services and operating costs by receiving a percentage of the worker's pay.

For example, the client pays the for-profit agency $12 an hour for a 40-hour week, which equals $480. The agency generally deducts *up to* 40 percent of the total for operating costs, Social Security, Medicare, taxes, and other amounts such as health insurance and local taxes. After deductions and taxes withheld, the worker is paid the balance of the $480. In this case, a total deduction of 40 percent would leave the worker with $288.

A not-for-profit home healthcare agency pays a set hourly, daily, weekly, or per-visit rate and collects payment from Medicare, Medicaid, insurance, or the client.

All home healthcare agencies have a minimum charge for a minimum visit of two to three hours. The minimum charge varies with the type of worker making the visit and hourly, daily, and weekly rates vary from state to state, from area to area. Higher rates will be found in places such as New York City and Long Island, New York; the Star Coast of California; Denver, Colorado; the Gold Coast of Florida, and in other densely populated areas. In rural areas, you may find rates considerably lower.

The pay rate chart below (for 1999) shows typical ranges of pay for domestic and home healthcare workers. Keep in mind your location and the skills of the particular type of worker you are seeking.

Type of Homeworker	Hourly wage Min/Max	Daily wage 8 hours	Daily wage 24 hours	Weekly wage 40 hours	Weekly wage live in
Home-maker	$5 to $15	$50 to $140	$75 to $160	$150 to $600	$250 to $700
Companion	$5 to $15	$40 to $120	$100 to $160	$150 to $750	$250 to $800
Home Health Aide	$5 to $20	$50 to $130	$80 to $240	$240 to $650	$260 to $900
Certified Nurses Aide	$7 to $25	$50 to $130	$130 to $280	$400 to $875	$500 to $950
Licensed Practical Nurse	$18 to $32	$140 to $260	$250 to $430	$600 to $1,000	$850 to $1,500
Registered Nurse	$25 to $60	$180 to $320	$480 to $680	$1,200 to $2,600	$2,500 to $5,000

These are ballpark figures, but at least you have a starting point. If possible, negotiate.

Healthcare agency pay rates are set and usually non-negotiable, but independent workers (those *not* hired through agencies) and those household workers placed by domestic staffing agencies, h/s/c agencies, and nurse registries can accept lower rates of pay, if they choose. An independent worker can be more flexible, depending upon working conditions and the volume of services the client will need.

Seldom will you find an R.N. or LPN working a live-in job. A client needing long-term, full-time skilled care will usually arrange for care outside the home.

When compared to hourly rates, live-in rates may seem skewed, but employers consider room, board, and perhaps the use of a vehicle as additional compensation to the worker. The worker, however, may see the live-in arrangement in a different light. A worker with a home and family may consider days absent as an inconvenience, not worth the extra "perks." A live-in arrangement might even include travel with the client which, depending on the worker, would or would not be a benefit. Live-in accommodations and travel plans should be clearly defined in a job description and, with the worker

DISCUSSED—DECIDED—PUT IN WRITING.

The term "live-in" has broad use. A live-in worker may stay in the client's home twenty-four consecutive hours and be on call only a fraction of those hours—say eight or twelve—and be free from duties the remainder of the day. Or the worker may stay on the premises twenty-four hours and be on call around the clock. Be certain to have a clear understanding with your homeworker of *hours on premises—hours on call.*

Randall, age 88

I had two full-time live-in aides. Beryl worked Monday through Friday, Linda worked the weekend.

Everything was fine to begin with. But after the first few weeks, Beryl got real short tempered. When I complained about her attitude, she explained. She hadn't understood, and I had failed to tell her, that I had a condition called nocturia, and that I needed assistance four or five times a night getting to and from the bathroom. She wasn't getting sleep and I kept her busy most of the day, not allowing time for her to rest at all.

We worked it out so that I would settle down every afternoon for a couple of hours, so she could catch up on her sleep. After we got that all worked out, her attitude changed and she was a lot more pleasant.

Before we leave the subject of the costs of care, let's look at three less well known sources of funds: long-term homecare insurance, reverse mortgages, and veterans' benefits.

Cost/Payment #7: Long-term Homecare Insurance

Until a few years ago, long-term care insurance covered only nursing home costs. Now more companies are writing policies that cover long-term homecare expenses. If you have this type of policy, have your agent explain in detail when and how much you can collect on your claims for homecare.

If you do not have long-term homecare coverage and you already have been diagnosed with a medical problem, chances are you will not be eligible for this type of coverage, or you will pay higher policy premiums.

If you need no medical or personal care—only companionship or custodial care at this time, you may want to investigate and insure for future long-term homecare.

If you decide to shop for long-term homecare insurance, consult at least three agents and read all written material carefully before making a decision. Here are some of the more important questions that you should ask about any plan:

- What is the **company rating** in *The Best's Insurance Reports Life / Health*? (Check in your library for this publication, or have your library research clerk check for you.)

- Is the premium **level for life**? (The policy may contain a clause that allows the company to raise premiums for *all* policy holders, and you will pay that increased premium.)

- Can the company **increase your individual premiums**, and for which reasons?

- Will the policy be **renewable for life**?

- Does the policy pay **homecare benefits**? And how does it pay—by a "dollar limit" or a "total days" limit?

- Is a **hospital or skilled nursing facility stay** required before benefits will be paid for homecare?

- Does the policy have a **waiver of premium**?

- Exactly what **dollar amounts** will the policy pay?

- Who determines the **need for homecare**—your physician or a physician appointed by the insurance company?

- What are your **appeal rights** if you do not agree with the insurance company on their "need for care" decision?

- After a need for care has been determined, is there a **waiting period** (elimination period) before benefits begin? If so, how long is that period?

- Is there an **exclusion** for **preexisting conditions**? If so, how long is that period?
- Does the policy cover **disability homecare**?
- Is the coverage for homecare only, or for homecare *and* nursing home care?
- Who decides the skill level of the care needed (HHA, CNA, LPN, R.N.)—you or the insurance company?
- If you are receiving Medicare benefits, will you pay for coverage of services that are already covered by Medicare?

For sources of additional, more in-depth discussion and information on long-term homecare insurance, check Appendix C.

Cost/Payment #8: Reverse Mortgage

If you have a condo or house that is paid for or has high equity, you may be able to arrange for a reverse mortgage on that property. A reverse mortgage is just one form of home-equity financing. You must talk to your banker, a mortgage broker, or a HUD representative to determine the amount of monthly payments you may qualify to receive. This money can pay for homecare you might not be able to afford otherwise.

As with most financial arrangements, there is a downside to the reverse mortgage. Possible long-term, ongoing care may erode all your equity, and you will face the risk of losing your home. Insist that the person you consult about this matter explains fully how a reverse mortgage is structured. Also be sure you get a "worst-case" scenario.

Cost/Payment #8: Veterans Administration

Military benefits, yours or your spouse's, may entitle you to certain homecare benefits from the Veterans Administration. Some V.A. hospitals and clinics have homecare units with which they work. Other outside private home-care agencies are not covered, except in a few cases when the veteran has a 50 percent or higher rated service-connected condition. This benefit is usually limited to recovery from a specific illness.

To determine if there is help for the veteran client, contact the Veterans Administration office. (See Appendix C for a main number. Check your phone book for a local listing.)

And now, on to Step Five: Interviewing and Soliciting Information. Take a few minutes first to get some fresh air, clear your head, and prepare for a heavy workout of your interpersonal skills.

6

Interviewing and Soliciting Information

As stated earlier in this section, if you hire a worker through most nurse registries, h/s/c agencies, or home healthcare agencies, the worker comes to you with an implicit guarantee of job suitability and client satisfaction, and you skip interviewing and go on to Step Six: Establishing and Maintaining a Successful Relationship With Your Homeworker.

One word of caution: If an agency sends a worker to your home and your "character instincts" act up or you feel an instant personality clash, speak with the agency supervisor as soon as possible. You are never obligated to accept a worker the agency sends to you. You, the client, are a customer and if you feel the worker is not suitable for you or your needs, you are not bound by the agency's decision to place a particular worker with you. Stay in close contact and communicate honestly with the agency supervisor. A good supervisor has advanced problem-solving skills and expects to use them.

Discussion in this chapter focuses on interviewing and obtaining information when you hire through a domestic staffing agency, classified ad, or an h/s/c agency—any source except a reliable personal reference or a home healthcare agency acting as a worker's direct employer.

If you hire through an agency, they will check references, personal background information, and professional credentials before the applicant arrives to interview. Depending upon state/federal requirements, the agency may also conduct a criminal check.

An established, reputable agency should do these things; however, not all established, reputable agencies take the time to complete paperwork and verifications on workers they send out. You and your advocate may want to check and verify information on your own. The worker you hire will have access to private areas of your home and your life, and you can never be too careful when selecting that homeworker.

In your first contact with an agency you also want to make your preferences in a homeworker known, and this might be awkward. Intending no discrimination, you may be fearful of people who look or sound different.

Estelle, age 92

I accept anyone to work with me and live in my home if they are honest and of good character. However, I have a dreadful time understanding heavy accents. This difficulty caused me and a West Indian woman who came to interview with me a most distressing experience.

During the interview, I barely understood what the woman was saying. I must say, she must have thought me daft.

I tried to explain my predicament to Mr. Moore at the agency, and he seemed sympathetic.

The worker I eventually hired was a woman from Paraguay who has a lighter accent that is, for me, easier to understand. We communicate well and everything is just fine.

If you are a woman, you may feel uncomfortable being attended by a male worker, or, believing that a man has greater strength for the physical requirements of a job, you may prefer a male worker. You cannot ask an agency representative to discriminate or to play favorites among registered workers, but you can ask that the representative help you establish a "comfort zone" with a homeworker. You may find yourself under unusual stress when seeking a homeworker. It is not a good time to analyze or attempt to cure fears that you or others may find inexplicable or unreasonable.

You, the client, hiring through a domestic staffing agency or a classified ad, will be wise to plan three stages in your hiring process. There are things you can do *prior to, during, and after the interview* to ensure a wise and informed hiring decision. Plan these three stages with your advocate, and, if hiring someone you already know, eliminate the parts of the process that you find unnecessary.

Prior to an interview, prepare a list of questions that you think are relevant. Ask them, and make notes about the applicant's responses. Be sure you have left adequate space after each question on your list in which to make notations: satisfactory answer, unsatisfactory answer, applicant hesitant, discuss further. Your list may include these questions:

- What do you like most about the work you do?
- Do you like animals . . . have pets?
- Are you looking for long-term or short-term employment?
- Are you willing to travel and spend winter or summer in a different location, if necessary?
- Do you have a résumé?

- Will you be available for extra hours, if needed?
- What type of transportation will you use to and from the job? Will your car be available for on-job use? If so, will there be a charge to me?
- Do you have your own health/liability insurance?
- Do you already have set plans that would necessitate that you have time off right away? (A worker may already have travel plans or appointments that they will not want to change. You should know about these plans up-front.)
- Will you give written consent for a background search and/or a personal handwriting analysis?

The last question may seem extreme, but this *is* a business arrangement and you must think of your safety and well-being. (Remember, it isn't *what* you say or ask, it's *how* you say or ask it.)

Next, arrange for your advocate to be present and set aside an adequate block of time for the interview. If you are rushed, you will conduct an ineffective and incomplete interview.

Make sure that the applicant has clear directions to your interview location, either from the agency or from you. Most often the interview is conducted in your home, so that you will be comfortable. This also helps the applicant get the feel of your environment.

Have the applicant, whether agency or independent, bring to the interview some form of photo identification and any professional licenses they hold. Be aware that in some states asking for a specific type of identification is against the law. After a person is actually hired, you are entitled to see one or two forms of official identification such as a Social Security card, a green card, or other ID that verifies the worker's right to work in the United States.

The second stage occurs *during* the actual interview. First, introduce your advocate to the applicant. Then, if you have received no résumé from an agency, ask the applicant if one is available. If not, provide pen and paper and ask that the applicant write full name (and maiden name, if applicable), complete current and former street address, Social Security number, closest relative not at same address, and a list of references.

If the applicant indicates that a recent client is deceased, ask for the name of the client's son, daughter, or another close relative as a reference.

With the applicant, go over the questionnaire you drew up previously, and be sure that your advocate feels free to ask additional questions.

The next step in the interview is to give the applicant a copy of your job description. See example, page 184. Just as you did with your questionnaire, have a copy of the job description on which you can make notes.

In the job description, you will have stipulated the duties you want performed. You will have been thorough, so there will be no surprises for the worker later. You will have made clear whether or not you will provide meals, and you will have set out a work schedule complete with meal and break times.

If you are hiring a live-in worker and your medical and physical condition permits, you will designate a daily two-hour "free" period for the worker. Agencies have been known to tell the homeworker that this free period is standard, yet neglected to inform the client of this fact, thus causing confusion at the very outset of the client/homeworker relationship.

Another point to cover in the job description is the worker's visitors on the job. The worker, especially if living in, may want friends and family members to visit.

You may want to limit those visits to the worker's immediate family members, limit the duration of visits, and limit visits to certain areas of your home.

If your worker has private quarters, you can be more flexible in your guidelines concerning visits. It's your call. If the worker lives in your main residence, you will want to consider the matter more carefully. If the worker is not agreeable to the guidelines you set forth, and the worker is the worker you really want . . .

DISCUSS—DECIDE—PUT IT IN WRITING!

You can include vacation time and pay rate in the job description to avoid clarifying the issue later. Customarily, after twelve months on the job, a live-in or weekly worker is due a one-week paid vacation.

For a live-in worker, consider allowing more frequent, shorter vacation breaks. Constant twenty-four hour interaction between you and a homeworker can become strained after a few months. In the job description, you can stipulate that you will pay for only one vacation period per year and leave the homeworker the option of taking additional time off without pay.

During the interview, observe body language. Eye contact is also important. "Shy" and "shifty-eyed" are not synonyms. There is also a difference between normal nervousness and nervous "fidgeting."

If possible, get written consent from the applicant to conduct a criminal or personal background check and/or a personnel handwriting analysis. Privacy laws are unclear in some states and you do not want to be accused of violating a worker's privacy. To secure permission to use these hiring tools, you need only say, "I hope you understand my concern. You seem to be a—nice, lovely, upstanding, decent (take your pick)—person, but I really need this extra peace of mind." If you will be uncomfortable with this part of the interview, let your advocate handle it.

Christopher, age 72

I'm getting a little shaky, so I decided to hire a valet. I started interviewing, and my daughter Jill helped me.

I've traveled all my life and collected artwork and artifacts worth a small fortune. I value many of these things for sentimental value reasons.

Therefore, I wanted all the peace of mind I could get. The gentleman I hired would have to have a reputation above reproach, perhaps not with his lady friends, but with other persons' property, and I was asking permission to run background checks of everyone who applied for the job.

The third applicant I interviewed was my choice for the job. However, when I asked for permission to do a background check, that gentleman called me a vile name, ranted about not being trusted, and slammed out of my home.

Jill and I were appalled. I almost felt ashamed for having asked him for such permission, but as Jill and I walked through the dining room, we paused to reminisce over a Dresden figurine my late wife had purchased in Europe. The memories were priceless.

My search for a valet took another two weeks, but I found an excellent employee. The background search on him turned up nothing untoward, and I have the extra peace of mind I was seeking.

If you don't know of anyone to run background checks for you, look in the Yellow Pages under Personnel Consultants or Private Investigators. Look under Handwriting Analysts, Graphology, or Graphologists to find a professional who, from a handwriting sample, can give you a personnel report. (See Appendix B.)

Always ask the applicant under which arrangement they will be working, independent contractor or employee? Remember to use IRS Form W-9, if needed. Discuss payroll period—weekly, biweekly, monthly—in detail with the applicant.

If you or your advocate feel the applicant is a strong possibility for hire (a subtle sign or a code word can signal agreement without your having to leave the room), you may want to give the applicant a brief tour of your home. If the applicant will be living in, show and discuss the worker's private quarters, and note positive or negative reactions by the applicant.

The third and final interview stage comes *after* the applicant has left the interview. While impressions of the applicant are still clear in your mind, go over your question sheet and job description with your advocate. Make additional notes and list additional questions you have for the agency supervisor or the applicant.

As soon as possible, pass on pertinent information to a personnel consultant or a private investigator for verification. Charges for services you contract from these professionals are quite reasonable. Usually for less than two hundred dollars and a wait of only two to three days, you should be able to obtain all the information and reassurance you need to help you make your hiring decision.

If you and your advocate check work references, ask each reference contact person how long the applicant held the job, ask what the job duties were, ask if those duties were performed satisfactorily, and ask if the applicant's termination happened under favorable circumstances.

After interviewing several applicants, checking references, and/or receiving information from the professionals you have enlisted, you are ready to make a final decision. If you have additional questions to ask an applicant, arrange a follow-up meeting. Also, if you are using a domestic staffing agency, verify the length of the agency's trial period, and stress to the applicant that you must know of any concerns that come up during that period.

You, the client, should be ready to do the same. Express to the worker any and all concerns you have during those initial few weeks. If you have undue difficulty establishing and maintaining clear channels of communication, you will terminate the relationship early on. If you take this action before an agency's trial period expires, you can save a great deal of money.

You have now completed the first five steps and have the necessary knowledge to find a homeworker suited to you and your needs. Now you are ready to go on to Step Six: Establishing and Maintaining a Successful Relationship With Your Homeworker.

7

Establishing and Maintaining a Successful Relationship with Your Caregiver/Homeworker

Learning to live with a new person in your life will be an ongoing adventure, bringing you new insights, not only about that person, but about yourself as well. As in any relationship, you will find there are issues to clarify, compromises to make, and delightful moments to share.

The guidelines for establishing and maintaining a successful relationship with any type of homeworker are the same, and this first one is crucial: Do not attempt to make the worker, or give the impression that the worker in your home is, "one of the family."

Why not? Because the relationship you have to maintain is a working relationship, not a familial one. Although the natural course in a home setting would seem to be that you, the client, and your worker become close very quickly, attempt to keep a professional distance.

Assume a friendly yet professional attitude toward a worker, and you will establish the foundation for a long and productive relationship. Still, the day may come when the relationship ends under less than congenial circumstances. If you have converted your caregiver or domestic worker to a family member, the separation will be emotionally painful and laced with unwarranted guilt.

Lillian, age 83

Angie kept the house spotless and indulged my every whim; I encouraged her to feel at home, and she did.

Once she became comfortable, she stayed up late to watch movies and got up late to prepare breakfast. Visits from her two grown daughters became quite frequent and soon included their small children.

Then I planned a trip to Switzerland. Angie immediately began planning what she would pack and arranged for her daughters to check my home while we were away.

When I managed the courage to tell her I was going alone, she protested. She told me I was ungrateful for all she had done for me. I apologized and tried to explain that I had wanted to be friendly and a good employer, but I had overdone it.

When I returned from Switzerland, I was lucky to find another woman to fill Angie's position. Again, I found myself slipping into that "too familiar" mode, but, believe me, I caught myself before I went too far.

As in any other type of job—office, factory, retail—professional distance is best kept between employer and worker. Do not make social occasions with your family or friends awkward because you feel you must include your worker. Be sure your worker understands and accepts the fact that you want to enjoy some or all of these occasions without the worker's immediate presence.

When you visit or dine out and want private time with friends or family, but need the assistance of your worker, make clear to the worker, in a respectful manner, when they should leave you. Direct the worker to an area to read, watch TV or shop until you need assistance. By setting distinct parameters of the client/homeworker relationship early on, you will be sidestepping potential problems. An ambiguous friend/business relationship can be confusing and destroy the objectivity you need when sorting out problem issues within a job setting.

As an example, you may encounter one of those few workers who, like untoward suitors, ingratiate themselves, endeavor to convince you of their indispensability, and take advantage of the close bond you have allowed to form. Remember to be wise, be aware, be a "friendly professional."

As a friendly professional, you show consideration and respect. If you have a complaint to air, by all means air it, but only after giving your cause for complaint deliberate thought. Look at a problem from your worker's point of view, then engage the worker in a calm, thorough discussion. Listen to and consider all that your worker has to say. If the issue is not personal, but job connected . . .

DISCUSS—DECIDE—WRITE OUT A SOLUTION

. . .then fill out and sign a resolution form.

Another point for you to consider: Be thoughtful of your homeworker by making your worker aware of, ahead of time, any variation in your daily schedule. You may have doctor, hair, or other set appointments that will break your normal routine. For you to give the worker notice of those activities is only fair. The worker can then plan the day more efficiently.

If you want special errands run, infrequently needed chores performed, or extra service of any kind, informing your worker in advance is a courtesy that costs you nothing.

There may be times when you, the client, feel you are not getting your money's worth from a homeworker. If you get that feeling, analyze the situation. Is the worker dodging chores, taking extra time for breaks and meals, cutting corners on household or healthcare responsibilities? If this is the case, then your resentment at paying full wages to the worker is justified. A meeting and discussion are called for.

If, however, your homeworker is performing all duties in the job description in a satisfactory and timely manner and, therefore, has extra time to relax and rest, allow the worker to do so. Keeping a conscientious worker busy every moment of the day by dredging up odds and ends of things to be done is not only inconsiderate, it is cruel. A worker is not a machine, but a person who can tire as the day wears on. Allow your worker a comfortable pace at which to work; you will derive no benefit if you wear down and burn out a worker who is doing a good job.

Respect a good worker's job efforts, and respect that worker's needs by:

- Honoring break times and allowing brief phone calls, business and personal.
- Allowing adequate time for unrushed meals—thirty to forty minutes.
- Introducing your worker to family and guests. Make the introductions short, but informative: "Natalie, this is my companion (nurse, homemaker, chauffeur)—Leslie. Leslie, this is my aunt (best friend, uncle, daughter, son)—Chris." The worker who is

professionally familiar with your circle of friends and family will be more efficient when taking or delivering messages for you.

- Keeping a "kitchen calendar". . . a calendar on which you notate appointments and plans that will include the homeworker.

- Saying "please" and "thank you," even though your worker is performing agreed upon tasks. These simple words from you will add an eager edge to a worker's job performance.

All of these considerations ensure a solid foundation on which your relationship with your worker will be built. One further note: Before you bring a worker into your home, you and a friend, family member, or advocate should double-check your home to make sure it is as accident proof as it possibly can be. Accidents can and do happen, and it is the client's responsibility to provide a safe work environment. Check your homeowner's policy for liability coverage and talk to your agent if you have doubts about your liability limit amounts.

Before you continue reading here, please read Chapter 19, On-the Job Needs/Live-In Arrangements.

Ray, age 95

When I hired nurses to look after me after my car accident (four nurses to cover twelve-hour shifts, seven days), I told them that I was retired military. I believe in schedule, routine, and order.

I made it clear they were not to have other people come into my home, but knowing they needed to keep in touch with their friends and families, I set rules for phone use.

On each twelve-hour shift, a nurse was allowed use of the phone four times and could talk for up to fifteen minutes—local calls, that is. They had to have calling cards for long distance calls, and I wanted incoming calls kept to a minimum. I preferred that they have pagers and return calls during regular breaks.

I allowed two fifteen-minute personal breaks and two meal breaks during each shift.

Others might not agree with my regime, but the people who worked for me knew when they started work what to expect, and believe it or not, I seldom had complaints of any sort.

If you have done your part, shown respect and consideration and discussed problem areas with a worker, and you find that the worker still is neglectful of assigned duties, you will want to dismiss that worker.

If at any time you feel uneasy with or intimidated by a worker in your home, something is wrong. Occasionally and unfortunately, a worker will develop a Boss Reversal Syndrome. You will recognize this syndrome when you hear the worker imply or say, "I know what I'm doing, don't bother me." Somehow, the worker has begun to take on the role of boss, *your* boss taking control of your home, your decisions, your daily activities.

The day a homeworker walks in and says, "I've got a headache, don't bother me," by all means, don't; just meet with your advocate to determine how soon you can replace that worker. (For more insight into the Boss Reversal Syndrome, see, page 174.)

"Pop-in" visits by friends, family members, and neighbors will help to keep a worker from assuming too much control. These impromptu visits alert your homeworker to the fact that the people in your life are concerned and interested in your well-being. Pop-in visits need not last long . . . just long enough for that second pair of eyes to look around and see that all is well.

Cynthia, age 52

I was out and about the other day, and decided to stop in and see how Mother was getting along with the aide she hired a few weeks ago.

Sitting down with Mother, I commented on the tantalizing food smells coming from the kitchen. Mother said, "It's Louise's cooking. She makes me a good home-cooked meal every night."

I wandered into the kitchen to say hello to Louise and compliment her on her culinary ambition. Louise was no where in sight. On the stove, boiling merrily away in a pot of beef broth, were two onions and a large stick of celery. On the counter was a Stouffer's frozen beef dinner.

It took me a minute to catch on. I opened the freezer and, sure enough, there was a week's worth of frozen entrees. How clever, I thought. I also wondered what other corners Louise might be cutting in her job-related duties—if they were extending to Mother's personal care.

Mother liked Louise, so Louise stayed, but I talked with both of them and increased the frequency of my unannounced visits.

So far in Step Six you have learned how to establish and maintain an effective day-to-day working relationship with a worker. You must also keep in mind practical matters such as bonuses and pay raises.

If your worker is from a healthcare agency, the agency will advise you about pay rate increases and Christmas and other bonuses.

If you have a direct employer/employee, client/homeworker arrangement, consider giving raises of 3 percent to 8 percent of gross pay per year. A Christmas bonus is a gift of appreciation for all the extra care and services your worker has provided you for the year past. Rule of thumb for this bonus is:

- lst year: one-half to one week's pay
- 2nd year: one to one and one-half week's pay
- 3rd year: At your discretion

You, the client, have no obligation to acknowledge a worker's birthday by giving a gift. You may use your own judgement. If you decide to give gifts, consider keeping them in the token, non-personal category.

Intimate knowledge of a worker's friends and family is another area you may want to avoid. As interesting as news from the worker's personal life may be, you may find that the worker wants to share more than you can tolerate. Since you will be in daily contact with your worker, discussions of a personal nature are inevitable. If you want to encourage these discussions, do so, but do not be surprised at what you may hear, and be sure to keep in place that "professional line" you have drawn for yourself.

Five or six months into the relationship you have established with your homeworker, you will realize that the manner in which you have adjusted to your role as client has been crucial to the success of that relationship. But you have adjusted, and the relationship is working.

The energy you and your advocate have expended on planning, research, and interviews has paid off. With loads of common sense and a little good luck, you will experience smooth sailing and have no further practical use for your newly acquired hiring skills.

If, by chance, you do need them in the future, take out this book (which you placed in a handy spot on your bookshelf), dig out your contact book and your files from your first search, call your advocate, and execute the process like a pro.

Take time now to read Section II for greater insight and understanding of the role your advocate will play in your homecare situation.

Then, to understand a homeworker's view of homecare, read Section III. By doing so, you will find that you, the client, will become effective beyond measure—a first-rate client/employer.

Ten Best Tips
for the Client

- **Arrange Pop-in Visits**. Have friends, family members, and neighbors stop in for frequent, unannounced visits.

- **When Hiring, Try to Find a Tag-team.** A tag-team is two or more workers who have worked together before, enjoy working together, and are willing to work for you as partners.

- **Ask and Investigate Everything!** Do not hesitate to ask as many questions as you can think of. Ask them of agencies, job applicants, organization representatives—everyone you encounter in your search for the best in homecare.

- **Keep Your Outlook on Life as Positive as You Can and Insist That Those Around You Do the Same**. A grouchy or negative-thinking worker, friend, neighbor, or family member can bring you down in a hurry. Tell them all to enter your home with an "up" attitude and keep it until they leave.

- **Be Flexible in Your Thinking**. Accept, to whatever extent you are able, new ways of making your life easier and new ways of solving problems.

- **Stay Open to Other's Opinions and Ideas**. If you don't like them or cannot accept them, you have at least kept an open ear; you haven't passed up good ideas by unequivocally shutting them out.

- **Acknowledge Your Own Vulnerability**. As difficult as it is to admit that you cannot manage daily activities as well as you once did, admit it, adjust, take care of what you can, and let others help you with the rest.

- **Trust Caregivers with Your Care, Trust Money People with Your Money.** Self-explanatory.

- **Put Yourself in Your Advocate's and Your Homeworker's Shoes.** Make an honest attempt to see your situation from their perspectives.
- **Talk, Talk, Talk.** Communicate often and explicitly with friends, family members—with anyone involved in your life. Let them know of your fears, your hopes, your problems, and your daily triumphs, both large and small.

BONUS TIP: Regardless of your physical or emotional condition, never wonder, "Why am I still here? What good am I?" As long as you are still breathing, you are still living. You have a purpose to serve, a place to fill. As long as you live, others will be learning from you—from your experiences, your pain (unfortunately), your triumphs, your cultural heritage, your love, your actions, and even your tears. All of these things about you carry lessons for others. As difficult as life may be for you, you remain here for a reason. Like it or not, you are a teacher.

SECTION II

The Advocate: The Assistant/ Helper

Responsibility is the thing people dread most of all. Yet it is the only thing in the world that develops us, gives us manhood or womanhood fibre.
Frank Crane

8

The Advocate's "Cause"

You've gotten the call: Help!

Who called? Your mother, father, a sister, brother, or friend, perhaps even a child.

You answer the call, listen to the plea: "I can't go any farther alone, but I want to stay at home. Can you find someone who will come here to help me?"

Perhaps you received no call, but you, or someone, has noticed changes in a person you care for and in that person's daily activities. Confusion, forgetfulness, depression, loss of appetite, crankiness, and physical frailty are just a few indications that a person may need homecare.

What type of homecare? Housekeeping chores, errands, personal care, and/or medical care. And why? Because of mental or physical frailty, loneliness, illness, or surgery aftercare.

And the reason that your friend or family member called you? Because, whether or not that person recognizes the term, they are in need of an advocate.

The word "advocate" as found in *Webster's New International Dictionary* has this meaning: "One that pleads the cause of another; defender."

The discussion here about advocates is not intended for the professional care manager or an agency case manager. The advocate who needs help, and lots of it, is the friend or family member who serves in this role.

If you assume the position of advocate, your "cause" will be the welfare and safety of the client, a person who is your friend or family member in search of either a domestic worker or a healthcare worker.

As an advocate, you will aid the client in locating, hiring, and living with a homeworker. You will serve as a buffer in all business conducted to that end.

If you are prepared to fill an exacting position, one which can bring unwarranted criticism and, often times, meager thanks, but sometimes abundant praise and gratitude; if you can be a cheerleader and protector of a person who, for whatever reasons, cannot stand up in his or her own behalf; if you can facilitate unfamiliar business with unfamiliar people in unfamiliar circumstances, then you can be a great advocate.

9

The Advocate: Family Member or Friend

The friend who serves as advocate and the family member who serves as advocate are very different in this one respect: the interaction each has had or will have with the client's family. A family member will probably feel more at ease discussing topics such as finances and personal health problems with the client than a friend of the client will. Then, too, perhaps not. In some instances, a family member and the client might share too much negative family history to discuss anything.

Vera, age 55

Stanley is an old friend of mine, and I was curious when his daughter Lila asked me to lunch.

"Dad needs someone to take charge," she said, "and it isn't me. He thinks I want his money. All I want is to get some help for him."

I knew that Stan, at the age of sixty, had suffered a second stroke. What Lila wanted was for me to be his personal manager, his advocate, and oversee his household and health interests.

I visited and talked with Stan several times. He finally confided in me that "Lila wants to spend all my money." I listened and reassured him as best I could.

As a trusted friend, I continue to help keep him calm and reassured. Lila is a sweet person and is very supportive of both her father and me.

Each client's homecare situation is unique, to be viewed by concerned parties according to its own special circumstances.

Regardless of your personal relationship to the client, be sure you make it clear that you are working *with*, not for, around, or over, the client. Take into consideration the client's mental, physical, and emotional ability to make decisions and take appropriate actions. If those abilities are limited, take more initiative, but be sure the person you are helping is acknowledged and feels respected. The situation the client is in is new and strange, and the client may feel threatened and humiliated. As advocate, you will give support, boost morale, and aid the client in practical matters.

So that you better understand how the client may feel, do this: *Change the client's face to yours, picture your home instead of the client's, then imagine having a stranger come to live with you.*

Mary Ann, age 35

Uncle Clint is my very favorite relative. He asked me to help him hire nurse aides and a homemaker after Aunt Eline got ovarian cancer, and I was real happy to do whatever I could.

Uncle Clint and I sat with Aunt Eline in her cozy kitchen and discussed her condition, the kinds of helpers she would need, and where we would find these people.

All of a sudden, Aunt Eline's voice, usually real soft, filled the room. "Would you like to ask *my* opinion, by any chance? I'm right here in the room, you know."

I felt really bad and I could tell Uncle Clint did, too. We shifted seats so Aunt Eline was looking directly across the table at me and Uncle Clint, just like she was the head honcho, which she was.

From then on, I asked Aunt Eline about every single thing I did that concerned her. As she put it: "It's my body that has a problem, not my mind."

There will be times as you go about your duties of advocacy when you will want to tell everyone where to go. You will have an occasional mad urge to jump an Asian-bound freighter or to stow aboard the next space shuttle. Please don't.

Instead, when you find yourself spending your last coin of patience, wherever you may be, excuse yourself. Find a quiet corner, a deserted hallway, an empty bathroom, and try to relax. Breathe deeply and use the projector in your head to run that picture of *you* in *your* home with a stranger, for one full minute.

Deb, age 41

I wanted to just strangle my mother. I was trying to help her but did she appreciate it? I didn't think so. It was bitch, gripe, and moan about her homemaker, the cook, the health aide who gave her range of motion, and even the kid who ran errands and did odd jobs for her.

I kept my cool until one day she started complaining that the cook had served the wrong sauce on the chicken. I almost exploded.

Holding back, I turned on my heel and stalked to the hallway bathroom where I gritted my teeth and muttered some very unpleasant things. For the longest, I stood looking out the window that faced the driveway.

Parked in the driveway was Mother's van with the wheelchair lift on the back. I lowered the toilet lid and, without the aid of the metal handle on the wall, sat down and did some thinking.

Before her stroke, Mother had been so independent, driving herself, doing for others. What must it feel like for her, in an instant, to have to depend on others? I tried to imagine.

These days, I'm more tolerant and I've encouraged her to work with a therapist who can help her overcome her frustration and depression.

Consider now the factors that may determine how full a role you will be able to fill as an advocate. The five main factors to consider are:

1. Whether you work, and if you do, your work schedule. The job you have may be too labor and/or time intensive for you to be effective in a role as demanding as that of advocate. You might be able to do good, but you also might do more harm than good. A tired, harried person can be a very impatient person.

2. Your relationship to the client. Your relationship with the friend or family member may be strained to the point that working and planning with that person is out of the question. Negative family history, grudges, or resentments will undermine the most well-intentioned efforts by both of you.

3. Your family and/or other caregiver/advocate responsibilities. You may already be buried under heavy responsibilities for your immediate family members: your wife, husband, children, and/or parents.

Renie, age 32
There were three of us kids who might have helped Dad when he got forgetful and feeble and couldn't look after himself, but none of us did it.

Well, we couldn't. I knew there was no way *I* could ever keep him going, and my brother Dinny is mean and ignorant . . . too busy with his girlfriends and racing buddies to do anything for anybody. And my sister Piquelle is a real airhead.

I do love Dad and I was scuffling to help. Turns out, I was real lucky. There was this nice woman at the health center who knew Dad and she offered to get help for him.

I made sure to tell her if it hadn't been for my five kids and having to hold two jobs, I would have done everything myself. I do what I can, but that woman was, and still is, a real life saver.

4. Your temperament. You may be lacking the temperament necessary to cope with the stresses involved in advocacy. Even if you deal with the most gentle-natured client, some of your "buttons" are going to get pushed. If you are short-tempered and impatient by nature, you should exclude yourself as an advocate. Instead, help the client by conducting a search for a person more suited for the job and once that person is found, give all the support you can.

Do not feel guilty because you cannot help as much as you would like, and do not be apprehensive because you cannot know every single minute what is going on with your friend or family member. Be realistic. All you can do is the best you can do, and that may mean that you will serve as a *subcontractor* advocate.

Acting as a subcontractor advocate, you can make calls and contacts, take notes, and relay information to the primary advocate. Volunteer, do what you can, when you can, but to avoid confusion, communicate all business directly to the main advocate, not to the client. The primary advocate will incorporate your information with other related information and present it to the client.

Channeling all information in this manner will keep it organized.

5. The distance you live from the client. If you live at an unhandy distance from the client, you will be restricted in the help you can offer, but there are a number of things you can do.

First, plan as long a visit as possible, then call the client's friends and family members who live close to the client and have them help you research by making calls to agencies and organizations. If you can't muster help in that manner, have the client or a friend send you a community services directory from the client's area and a telephone book, so that you can make the calls yourself. If you are interested in hiring from newspaper classified ads, have the client send you a Sunday paper or, if you live in a large city, purchase from a newsstand a paper that comes from the client's area.

Using these resources, have brochures mailed to you and the client. Call and set up appointments with employment agency supervisors and the client's doctor. Check classified ads and make preliminary calls to prospective workers.

When you arrive in the client's area, you can schedule interviews, hire the homeworker(s) needed, and observe them in the client's home.

Arrange for family members and friends, whether at a distance or close by, to make daily telephone calls to monitor the client's welfare. Or check out a large electronics store like Best Buy for a Via-TV or a modular video phone system. The cost of these systems runs from $800 to $1,500 (includes both the calling and receiving ends). If you can afford one of these systems, the peace of mind it will bring is well worth the cost. When you are many miles away, being able to actually see that the client is well and content will give you much-needed peace of mind.

If money is available, you can help the client hire a *professional care manager* to take care of everything. (Read about care managers in Section I, pages 31–32.) However, you will still want to meet the care manager and make your own assessment of that professional's capabilities.

Keep in touch with the client and encourage the client to call you and friends and family members often. If phone calls to you become excessive, or if the client calls at odd times of the night, check to make sure that everything is stable within the homecare situation.

Also stay alert for changes in tone of voice or mood that indicate that the client may be troubled. A client may hesitate to "bother" you with a problem, but a problem in a homecare setting, no matter how small it may seem, can become an enormous problem. A problem needs to be identified as soon as possible, even if you have to nag the client to get information.

Consider carefully the five factors you have just read. If one or any combination of those factors apply to you, you may want to exclude yourself as an advocate.

With the information and options given to you in the previous paragraphs and other information that only you know about yourself, you have made a decision—or are ready to make a decision—about taking on the role of advocate. Explore all the ramifications that advocacy has for you, then, if you decide to give it a go, give it all you've got.

You have decided. Now it's time for action. Where do you go from here? For starters, you will support the client's decision to set up homecare. Then you will help the client research, network, and interview to find a suitable worker. After the search is over and the worker is settled into the household, you will establish and maintain a compatible relationship with that worker; you will also be there to help settle any problems that arise between the client and the homeworker.

That you are supportive of the decision that the client has made is, of course, vitally important. If you think that a nursing home, an assisted living facility, or the home of a relative might be a wiser or more practical choice than homecare, discuss your thoughts in a conversational tone with the client. If you sound disapproving, your comments will add to the frustration and apprehension that the client may already be feeling.

Put yourself in your friend's or family member's situation. If that person has reached the point of admitting the need for help, the realization that day-to-day life will never be the same has already had a significant impact that has to be unsettling. Judgmental or antagonistic comments will only disconcert the client further.

David, age 50

"I'm not going to a home of *any* kind, and that's that." My father glared at me. "You're a writer. Go write. Leave me alone."

He was having one of his more lucid moments. His Alzheimer's was allowing few of these, and I wanted to take advantage of this one. I wanted to talk to him about his going to an Alzheimer's facility.

Not that he couldn't afford to stay at home and hire aides who could keep him from hurting himself or wandering out onto Fifth Avenue in the middle of traffic. He could very well afford anything he wanted.

But aides kept burning out and leaving. My sister and I were weary of the stream of white-uniformed men and women in and out of Father's place. *We* were the ones who listened to their complaints and found replacements.

Sis, Father, and I went round and round. Time and again, Sis and I upset Father and then had to calm him down. What torture we put ourselves through before we finally realized he was entitled to live wherever he pleased.

When we faced the fact that Father's care was going to be a full-time job, Sis quit her job and took on the supervision of his care. For the three years until Father died, Sis went through exquisite hell, but Father stayed where he most wanted to be.

Be understanding, be respectful, be all the help you can be. Read Section I, then using the information you find there, you can begin your search for a suitable home-worker for the client . . . you can start researching and networking.

10

Researching and Networking

Before you make the first phone call on behalf of the client, agree with the client on a method of documenting information. Keep files on everyone you contact and everything you learn.

You can assemble a simple but effective filing system by using colored spiral notebooks. Label them with a big tip, black marking pen: Medicare, Private Insurance, Personal Financial Papers, Interview Material, Employment Agencies, Neighborhood Resources, Health History Information, and Miscellaneous. Write important phone numbers on the front of each folder.

Another effective filing system can be set up using clear file folders, open on top and right side, found in office supply stores. The first page of your files can be easily seen and, again, important phone numbers can be written on the front of the file.

When making phone calls to gather information, have at hand the client's files and personal information including Social Security number, medical records, and financial papers. Also, have your list of questions ready.

When you are on a call on behalf of the client, you may be told by the person on the other end of the line that you cannot give or receive certain information. In that case, put the client on the phone, so that the client can continue the conversation or give permission for you to do so.

When calling for information, remember to:

- Note the date of the call.
- Ask for the name of the person you are speaking to.
- Ask clear questions.
- Insist on clear answers.
- Do not let yourself be rushed off the phone.

Although getting correct information is time and energy intensive, it is better that you get correct information at the outset of your research than to have to make callbacks.

Following are several valuable tips for researching on the telephone.

Do not make calls immediately before you have errands to run or appointments to keep. Without fail, you will be on the phone longer than you expect.

Call as soon as a company or agency opens. As the day wears on, nerves fray (yours and theirs), calls pile up, and patience dissipates.

If your requests for information are futile, ask for a supervisor or hang up and call back; sooner or later, you will get someone who is willing to help.

If you have been reasonable and pleasantly assertive in your attempts to gain information and still have nothing—cry. Cry for real or pretend to be having a nervous breakdown. The most frigid clerk melts upon hearing sobs, then the plea: "Please help me . . . I just don't know what to do . . . I've tried everything . . . I can't find out anything . . . Oh, please . . ." etc., etc., etc.

Prepare to listen to endless topic menus and relax (yes, relax!) by having a snack and beverage at hand, other paperwork you can do, your favorite music or TV show on, or interesting reading matter within reach. After listening to "Press one, press two . . ." and finally being put on hold for twenty minutes, you deserve those pleasant diversions.

If you use a speaker phone, you can roam the room, exercise, or dust while you wait for a real person to come on the line. A portable phone will extend your movement to the kitchen, bathroom, or balcony. Just be sure you can get back to your files quickly without interrupting an important activity.

Sandra, age 28

When I was trying to get Mom grooved in at home, there were, like, a zillion things to do. Like making all those phone calls. And, just no one would ever be there in person—menus, voice mail, recordings were all I got. I was trying to make a living working at home as a Web-site designer and I didn't have time for all that nonsense.

My friend Tracy is a super-freak organizer. She's married and has a kid, so I guess she has to be, and she came to my rescue like Wonder Woman.

She pulled a utility desk out of the garage and right-angled it to my computer desk. In, like, just a few minutes, she had file folders labeled, a speaker phone on one side of the desk and a portable phone on the other. She put a TV tray to the right of the desk and that's where she put a covered dish of my favorite snacks and a bottle of Evian water. She even set up a Rolodex with all those numbers I had scattered from here to forever.

Calling around for Mom was pretty cool after that. I did have one problem: trying to remember who I was calling when a warm body finally got on the other end of the line. I learned to write the name on a sticky note and put it on the desk in front of me to jog my memory.

If all attempts to gain information over the phone from a business or an organization have been unsuccessful, take the time to go to a physical location near you and, if possible, talk to someone nose to nose. To do this may require several hours of your time, but again, correct information is absolutely essential to the client's decision making. (For Medicare and Social Security information call the number listed in Appendix C.)

For information about hiring a homeworker, consult your local Yellow Pages and call businesses under the headings of Nurses, Healthcare Agencies, Employment Agencies, Geriatric Care Managers, Private Care Managers, Home Health Services, Social Service Organizations, Hospice, and Volunteer Organizations.

Have brochures and forms mailed to you and your client. You, the advocate, will be wise to set up your own information file, a file you can keep without inconveniencing the client. You can use that file to research away from the client's home.

Once you have gathered adequate information on finding a homeworker, you can start networking.

The wider you "spread the net" when you make your telephone and personal contacts, the more information you will have to work with. In Section I, the client was advised to draw up a Need List to help determine the type of homeworker needed. As you go through the files of sources from which you will draw, refer to that list.

Networking to cover all of the client's needs, bring all your sources together. Remember to call organizations such as the local Area Agency on Aging, the American Association of Retired Persons, and the community services center.

Katie, age 58

My mother was ninety-nine and completely bed-ridden. She had no particular illness, she was just very frail. She didn't sleep well, she was always restless and wanting to talk, wanting the bed-pan—she just wanted someone to be there.

I have brothers and sisters, but I was the only one free of responsibility and in good enough health to oversee Mother's care. With limited resources, I had to be extra creative.

I stayed with Mother during the day, and I found a retired aide who sat with her at night. My nephew ran errands and picked up meals from a local restaurant when I was too tired to cook and our wonderful neighbors dropped by with food from time to time.

I called the Area Agency on Aging and was put in touch with volunteer agencies that could provide someone to relieve me for a few hours each day. I also called the Children of Aging Parents organization; they gave me a lot of referrals and helpful information.

Mother lived until she was 102. Sometimes I thought I would go before she did, but with the wonderful help I had, I made it.

As you network, use your imagination and consider sources of help other than the "normal" ones. If you need transportation and taxi service is unreliable in your area, call a limousine service. Often an hour's rental or a trip to the doctor will cost little more from a limo service than it will from a taxi service. You can also call a friend or church member who has a car and possibly several hours to volunteer.

For help with meals, coordinate friends and family members to drop off prepared meals or special dishes several times a week. Query restaurant cooks and private chefs about preparing and packaging precooked or ready-to-cook meals.

Friends and family members can help you by shopping and running errands. They can pick up staple items for the client while shopping for their own groceries. This cuts down in-store time for the client and the homeworker. Recruit a young person, a friend, or a family member to pick up dry cleaning and prescriptions, perform household chores, and oversee automobile maintenance.

Enlist as many family members and friends as possible to help keep the client busy and entertained. Have everyone encourage the client to remain involved in club and church activities and to pursue entertainment interests they have always had.

If the client is unable to stay busy independently, check out adult day care and respite care. Adult day care is usually found at senior centers, community centers, and in some nursing homes. This service is for those adults who need activity and involvement but who do not need personal care.

Respite care provides monitoring of personal care and companionship for clients, so that primary caregivers can take breaks from their regular, stressful routines. These breaks are of great benefit to the client, as well. At a center, or even at home, respite care consists of some or all of these activities: exercise programs, social activities, information sessions, educational programs, and recreational activities. Because respite care is sponsored by community organizations, it is provided at low cost and is sometimes even free.

Explore all the above networking possibilities and set in place the assistance you find within them. If you find that additional help is needed, you and the client must turn to professional sources.

As you explore professional sources—newspaper classified ads and various agencies—you need to know how to conduct a successful interview, one which gives you the vital information you need to make the best possible choice of a homeworker.

11

Interviewing and Gathering Applicant Information

If you and the client have found a worker through personal recommendation, you will have background information on the worker and need only to arrange an informal "getting-to-know you" interview. If this is not your scenario, you and the client must make worker contact through some other source—a domestic staffing agency, a nurse registry, a healthcare agency, or a classified ad.

If you have decided to work with an agency, have a director or supervisor visit the client's home to draw up a care plan and set up interviews for you with several applicants. Let the director or supervisor know which days and times will be convenient for you and the client to hold interviews.

If you are going to hire through newspaper classified ads, select several ads, then call and ask questions over the phone (pre-interviews) to determine if you want to follow up with in-person interviews.

Before you schedule an interview, be prepared to conduct one that is well planned, one that will provide you with enough information to carry out thorough background checks and make a decision.

To prevent confusion and interview overload, interview only one type of worker—cook, chauffeur, healthcare worker, or homemaker—on any given day, and limit the number of interviews to no more than three a day if your hiring deadline permits.

> ### Ken, age 48
>
> I spent my vacation looking for a companion/homemaker for my parents who are in their eighties and unable to keep themselves or the house. I contacted several healthcare and staffing agencies to ask about pay rates and to see if they had workers available. After the first week, when I thought I was ready to start interviewing, I had no idea who was who or where to start. The notes I had made were pretty rough and scattered.
>
> After spending two days getting organized, I was determined to stay that way, so when I did set up interviews, I made a point to interview applicants for companion one day and applicants for homemaker on another day. I knew if I mixed them up I'd be confused all over again. I never dreamed that something that seemed so simple, hiring a couple of people, could be so involved.

You, the advocate, should always be with the client during interviews. If you cannot be present, arrange for another person to sit in for you. Whoever is with the client during the interview will have antennae out, feeling for reassurance in these four areas:

- Is this applicant trustworthy; will the client be safe with this person?
- Will this applicant be a competent, efficient, and conscientious worker?
- Will this applicant be compatible with the client? In demeanor, is this person too frenetic, too aggressive, or too shy?

- Is the applicant self-centered? Is this person talking about the client's interests, or about self-interests?

Pay close attention to the general demeanor of the applicant and trust your instincts when assessing your overall impressions.

During the interview listen intently, make notes, and ask questions that the client may not have thought of. Observe the applicant for cleanliness, politeness, and show of interest. Also observe if the applicant is open and compliant when answering questions.

Helen, age 65

When my friend Charlotte had to hire permanent help after her bypass surgery, I offered to help. I'd do anything for her. I helped her interview then, and I'm still helping her now when interviews come up. Charlotte says she feels better if I'm at the interviews with her.

I always think of questions she forgets to put on her question list. Just like the time Charlotte was ready to hire an aide right on the spot.

I thought to ask, "Do you have transportation?"

The woman said, "Yes, my husband will get me here, except on Thursdays I will be coming at ten instead of eight in the morning, and then on Mondays I have to leave early, because of his second job."

I started to speak, but she continued. "Oh, and I may bring my granddaughter sometimes. My daughter's baby-sitter takes time off every once in a while."

If I hadn't thought to ask that one question, I'm sure Charlotte and I would have been looking for another aide within a very short time.

Unless the client has asked that you be in charge, allow the client to conduct the interview. If the client decides during the interview that an applicant is a possible hire and wants to show that applicant around the home, accompany the client and applicant on the tour. Be unobtrusive and discreetly observe the applicant's demeanor. Is the applicant reasonably relaxed and interested in what the client has to say? If there are pets in the home, is the applicant at ease with them? Does the applicant ask pertinent questions about daily routine, private space, and the client's personal preferences within the home?

When the interview and tour are over, ask additional questions you may have. One such question, if the applicant has made a favorable impression, is "If (client's name) wants to hire you for this position, when are you prepared to start?"

In Section I, the client was advised to have background checks run on possible hires. As advocate, you will help the client eliminate those applicants that you and the client agree are unsuitable for the job, then you will help the client decide about running criminal and/ or background checks on the remaining candidates.

If you decide to run background checks, locate a private investigator or personnel consultant who is knowledgeable about privacy laws in your state. (If you have no personal referral or recommendation, check the Yellow Pages to find either of these professionals). Of course, you will make the applicant aware that you are going to conduct a background check and you will get written consent to do so.

A personnel evaluation executed by a handwriting analyst can be a valuable hiring tool when you are attempting to decide which applicant is best suited to the client's needs. A graphological evaluation can give insight about a potential worker's patience, like or dislike of detail work, ease of relating to other people, practicality, and general intelligence.

Handwriting analysis is a behavioral science (designated so by the Library of Congress), and has been used as a support hiring tool in some departments of companies like Olsten Corp. and Citibank. (Refer to Appendix C for a select few handwriting consultants. Check your local Yellow Pages for others.) As you did with the background check, make sure the applicant is aware that you may use this type of hiring aid and get written consent to do so. Assure the applicant that there is nothing psychic or "spooky" about handwriting analysis; it just shows clearly basic character traits.

The more information you have about a worker who is coming into the client's home for the first time, the more confident you will feel. Information from an objective source can verify and supplement your own information. This is reassuring, as the client's safety and well-being are your basic concerns and of the utmost importance. You never want to have regrets about a decision that you made, or helped to make, which ultimately endangered a friend or family member.

Ernestine, age 60

From the interview and the résumé that this particular job applicant had given us, I was ready to hire her as Father's companion/homemaker as soon as the interview ended.

But my eighty-year-old father is a deliberate and cynical man. He let her go, and then called a private investigator and had him run a background check. He also had the woman's permission for a handwriting analysis and ordered one.

The results? The background check revealed that she was listed under ten Social Security numbers,

> that she had moved three times in the last year,
> and that her driver's license had been revoked.
>
> The handwriting analysis showed she was highly
> intelligent, but tended to be impatient, and that
> she was overly emotional and not given to com-
> promise. All in all, not a good candidate to work
> with Father, who is as stubborn as they come.
>
> We continued the search, getting permission each
> time for checks and analysis. It took a full month,
> but we found a man who has proven to be a great
> worker who is perfectly compatible with Father.

The client may take an instant liking to and feel comfortable with a particular applicant, and you may feel
the same. If you and the client are not able to make a
quick decision, however, sorting-out sessions are in order.

Together, go over all the information you have on
your most likely prospects. Determine if there is one applicant who seems most suitable for the client's needs. If
you find that none of the applicants is suitable, you will
begin a new series of interviews.

Eventually, much wiser than when you began the
interview and hiring process, you will find a homeworker
who fits the client's needs satisfactorily.

12

Establishing and Maintaining Your Role as Advocate

That your enthusiasm and confidence about the worker you hire will be put to the test (and probably more than once) is a certainty. Before the homeworker reports for the first day of work, that worker, the client, and you, the advocate, will have agreed upon a trial adjustment period. This period should be a generous one that lasts four to eight weeks.

By the end of that trial adjustment period, you and the client will have arrived at a certain level of comfort with the worker. Or not.

Becoming *fully* at ease with and accustomed to a worker takes three to six months. During that time, your goal as advocate is to establish a relationship of mutual respect and trust with the homeworker. In establishing that relationship, you want to communicate openly. You want to be patient. And you want to be assertive, not demanding, in your position of authority.

As an effective advocate, you must wear many hats. You are *surrogate* and *protector* for the client and *mediator* and *sounding board* for both the client *and* the worker.

As surrogate for the client, you will make stressful decisions and take action when events become overwhelming for the client.

Janette, age 36

Two weeks after I helped Mom and Dad hire a home health aide, I got a fretful call from Mom.

"Jan, hon, this woman has got to go. She's moving all my things around. Right now, I don't know where anything is."

I made the trip from Orlando back down to Delray Beach to look in on the folks. Sure enough, the overly efficient home health aide had rearranged the contents of all the kitchen cabinets, bathroom cabinets, and bureau drawers.

I couldn't argue the fact that the pots and pans were neat when sorted to size; that the salt and pepper shakers were handy right above the stove, and that Mom's undergarments arranged bra/girdle, bra/girdle looked very nice. But Mom and Dad were lost.

I discussed the matter with the aide, who looked at me as if I were crazy. She said, "I just can't work in a disorganized environment."

I talked her into trying, but after another few weeks, we all agreed to an amiable parting. To be sure, when interviewing for a replacement, even though the folks were reluctant to bring up the subject of obsessive-compulsive behavior, *I* made sure to watch out for any applicant who gave a hint of it.

Filling the role of the client's protector, you will guard against those unscrupulous professionals who bully, deceive, and take advantage of trusting, vulnerable people, old and young alike. Sad, but true, is the fact that there are those domestics and healthcare workers who lack the ability to empathize with their clients.

Antony, age 62

I pop in on Mama a few days after I find the just right woman for her. I come to make a nice surprise for lunch. And when I see her there, I am angry.

Mama is to eat with a bib around, and she looks sad at a plate with greens. Bottles lined in front of her with lots of pills—"vitamins." That woman say to me, "Your mama wasn't eating good, but I fix her up."

Fix her up? I leave that woman to clean up and I take Mama to Mario's. Over a plate of pasta with the good red sauce, Mama tells me how the woman make her eat the different food, how she tell the woman no. The woman treat Mama like a baby, she tell Mama she don't know good food to eat.

I keep my anger, but when we get home, I send Mama to nap. Then I tell the woman, "You leave now," and I pay her money. I don't think twice. I send her away.

Again I look for a nice lady who cook Mama good pasta and vegetables. But now? Me and my wife, Rosa, we see that Mama is happy.

Often, workers don't realize that they are bullying. Ask and they will tell you, "I am only doing what is best for my client." Homeworkers, especially caregivers, work closely with the client, and their perspective can become skewed; their priorities misplaced. If you, the advocate, notice inappropriate use of control and authority by a homeworker, be sure to talk to the homeworker and get the balance of control and authority readjusted in favor of the client.

Also as protector, you will watch and listen closely, making certain that the client is not given to unreasonable generosity to homeworkers.

When it comes to gifts and giving, some clients are more vulnerable than others. There are those who can say no when asked for a loan of either money or property. When a worker casts a wistful eye and offers compliments on a pretty trinket or treasured collectible, there are clients who can just say thank you, and leave it at that. Others can not.

As a conscientious advocate, stay watchful for items missing from their usual places. Inquire of the client about missing items. This is not nosiness on your part, it is justified concern. Someone needs to know. The client has a right to dispose of property, but should not be under duress when that disposition is made. And if the client chooses to give away expensive items or family heirlooms, be wise and inform a close family member. Let that family member bring up the subject to the client, so that the absence of the items can be acknowledged.

These actions on your part will protect you, the advocate, in the event of the client's confusion or death, from questions regarding the whereabouts of particular items that may be missing from the client's home.

As mediator and sounding board, you will receive complaints from both the client and the homeworker. You will temper their separate approaches to a problem when both of them have valid points of view. If the client cannot cope with problems, make certain that the homeworker feels free to come to you with questions and concerns.

When disagreements or misunderstandings arise about time off, duties not performed, incorrect pay figures—anything at all in the client/homeworker relationship—listen to both sides and clarify the information you receive. Then write out the salient points of the dispute and a proposed resolution to the problem, and fill out a resolution form like the one found on page 24. Or, if the client prefers to cope with the problem and handle the resolution with the worker, let the client do so. Just be sure that the problem is . . .

DISCUSSED—DECIDED—PUT IN WRITING.

Be sure that the client follows through by having a resolution form signed and filed for future reference.

CiCi, age 48

Mother isn't, never has been, the most adorable person to live with. I can say that because I just do absolutely dote on her. But she was totally naive when she hired a live-in companion for the first time. Everyone here uses Tupper's Agency, and they sent Mother a top-drawer lady to send out Mother's notes, answer her telephone, and do all those nuisance things that just must be done.

Oops, though. Mother just did lose her dignity one day after luncheon, when Vita (Mother's companion) insisted on having two hours off for herself.

Well, whatever did I know? I called Michelina at the agency, and she said, "All of my live-in workers get two-hour daily breaks. Didn't I tell you?"

I explained to Mother, "We didn't know now, did we? You aren't absolutely dying or anything, Mother. Do send Vita out. Late afternoon, during your rest, is a perfect time."

Mother grudgingly agreed. Vita was thrilled. I was relieved, absolutely.

Mediation may be necessary when a problem arises between two homeworkers. Your best approach is to speak to each worker privately, sort out the problem for yourself, then discuss with the workers the resolution you think best and implement it. Again you will be . . .

DISCUSSING—DECIDING—PUTTING IT IN WRITING.

Andrea, age 57

Dad's health-aide, Eve, had been with him six years; she was overbearing at times, but she was good to Dad and I liked her.

Then Dad fell, and as part of his rehab, he worked with a physical therapist twice a week. While the therapist worked with Dad, I would take a rest. It was during the therapist's sixth visit that Eve came pounding on my door.

"Andrea, you tell that idiot that Mr. Coile is finished for the day, and that's that."

I followed Eve into the living room, where she promptly wheeled Dad away to his bedroom out of the sight and hearing of me and the therapist. I soothed the therapist, and showed him out.

Later, Eve and I sat and talked with Dad. Eve said the therapist had insisted Dad keep walking even though Dad had told him he felt he was going to fall. Dad also confided that the therapist had been, at times, rough when handling him. Dad, looking apologetic, said, "Seems like he didn't like fooling with me."

I called the agency supervisor, and they sent out a different therapist. I asked Eve to let me know right away in the future if she sensed a problem.

After being an advocate for a while, you will have become, in a sense, a "resolution specialist." The client/homeworker relationship you will have witnessed is unique—a relationship that has to exist on a personal/impersonal level, a delicate situation, indeed, and you will be right there in the middle of it. With all your patience, perseverance, and peacemaking skills, you will find yourself wondering *what the heck am I doing here?*

To help you through those moments of travail and doubt, contemplate the "thinking points" listed in Self-care for the Advocate.

13

Self-care for the Advocate

Frayed nerves, low energy, frustration overload. Serving as an advocate, sooner or later, you will experience those three maladies, and more.

Go through the six thinking points listed here. Follow up on these points, and they will help to push you over the exhaustion bumps you may hit. Think these points through when you begin your advocacy, and rethink them often as you serve in that capacity.

1. Be good to yourself.
You are special. You are doing something that not many people will or can do. Give yourself a pat on the back, a mental hug. Look in the mirror and say, "Thank you. You are doing just fine." In the normal course of events, you will seldom hear that acknowledgment from anyone else. Everyone is busy these days, living at a pace so breakneck, they will have little presence of mind to thank you.

2. Don't be a martyr.
Remember: You have the option of recruiting someone else to be the client's advocate. If you find yourself thinking or saying, "How unhappy I am. But I have to do it. No one else will. What a burden," the person you are trying to help is going to be aware of your weariness. Your

heaviness of spirit will make the client feel worse in an already difficult situation. If you find that you do not get a bona fide sense of satisfaction from aiding someone in need, don't do it. An act performed with underlying resentment carries with it negative feelings, negative vibrations. And it can, and almost certainly will, make you sick, if not in your spirit, then in your mind, and if not in your mind, then in your body and perhaps in all three. Act long enough with underlying resentment, and you will be a pitiable human being, of little good to anyone, including yourself.

3. Conserve your energy.
Make a list of people who can help you to help the client. Think of ways to give yourself "rest stops," as you go about your advocacy duties. Take a twenty-minute walk, take a coffee break, go alone into a room and listen to your favorite music, or find a quiet spot and read a passage in a favorite book. Give yourself a gift, a moment of freedom from responsibility.

4. Set your priorities.
Be realistic. Can you—will you—be effective as an advocate with the time and attention you have to give? No? Don't beat yourself up, because you cannot place advocacy at the top of your list. Instead, allot wisely the time and attention you *can* give. Constantly remind yourself that at the top of your priority list, there is room for only *one* person, one activity. That's just the way it is.

5. Love or money: why you serve.
Will being an advocate bring you money? Will it bring you love and affection? Could it possibly bring you both money *and* love and affection?

If your interest in the client is fed by a monetary incentive—benefiting from the client's assets, receiving special monetary favors, being named as beneficiary in a will—be honest with yourself about that, then keep your peace, and be the best advocate you can be.

If your interest is fed by the need for affection from the client, all you can do is hope that you will receive that affection, someday, somehow. But you cannot count on it. Face the painful fact that the affection you want may never be forthcoming, then look upon the client as simply a person in need and be the best advocate you can be. Do that for yourself. At least you will have the satisfaction of knowing you did all you could, aware all the while that you might never get what you wanted. Believe it or not, that can be a good thing.

6. Someday *you* may be a client.

This final thinking point is due long and deliberate contemplation. As you read this, you have reached a certain age and you may be in excellent health. You may have money, property, fame, and adoration; your life and your loves may be charmed. And you may keep all these wonderful things for many years to come, but there are two things you cannot keep—youth and perfect health. You are slowly, but surely, growing older.

Will you need help someday? Will you need an advocate? Will you need someone who cares—someone to give you care? Perhaps you will, and your acceptance of the fact that you may reach that point in your own life will, perhaps, motivate you to help others now.

Occasionally remind yourself that you will always have priorities to set, emotional hurdles to overcome; however, be a helper when you can.

If you hit a spell of weariness and the thinking points aren't spurring you on, take an uninterrupted break of several days away from the client. Arrange for others—

respite care, adult day care, friends, and family—to take over the chores you have been handling. Explain to the client that, barring an extreme emergency, you will be unreachable—that you have matters to which you must attend. You have no obligation to reveal to the client what those matters are.

The client may not realize how stressful your position as advocate is, and that you need an occasional break to enable you to continue in that role. The client may not understand if you try to explain that you need several days to recharge your battery, refresh your perspective, and regain your sanity. Explaining the reasons for your "recess" may be unproductive and cause consternation and resentment from the client. Just take your break, enjoy it, then carry on.

You may need these breaks often. Take them and refuse to feel guilty. Keep in mind that an exhausted, burnt-out advocate is of no good to anyone.

This section was not written to discourage those of you who would serve as advocates. It was written to offer you survival tips and to aid you in making decisions and preparing for the educational and enlightening role you are thinking of taking on.

For an eye-opening view of homecare from the caregiver's perspective, read Section III, The Caregiver: Friend, Family, or Professional. You will gain valuable insights and discover tools you can use when serving as liaison between your client and the homeworkers who become a part of the client's life.

Ten Best Tips
for the Advocate

1. **Do Not Assume That You Know What is Best for the Client.** Listen to the concerns, ideas, and fears of the client with whom you are working. Instead of dictating what you think should be done, be sympathetic, empathetic, and offer suggestions.

2. **Talk *to* the Client, Not Past, Around or Through the Client and Insist That Others Do the Same.** Even the longtime physician of the client may be guilty of discussing the client in the third party, as if the client cannot hear or speak in his or her own behalf.

3. **Accompany, or Have Another Responsible Person Accompany the Client to All Medical Appointments.** Paperwork, instructions, and follow-up information can be overwhelming for a client, and the presence of a supportive second person is usually welcomed.

4. **Marshal the Troops.** Network and plan. Call on everyone you can think of to help fill the needs of the client.

5. **If Possible and If the Client Will Permit, Have a Professional (CPA or Accountant) Handle All Household Bills and Payroll.** Do not ask homeworkers or inexperienced friends or family members to coordinate the client's financial affairs.

6. **After a Homeworker Has Been Accepted into the Client's Household, Support That Worker as Best You Can.** Keep communication flowing, and encourage the worker to confide in you about all work-related matters and even personal conflicts with the client. You need to be aware if trouble is brewing about *anything*.

7. **Make Pop-in Visits.** Make these visits and arrange for others to make them, also. Stay alert for unnatural or troublesome activity of any kind in the client's household.

8. **Never Jump to Conclusions When Hearing One Side of a Client/Homeworker Problem.** Be diplomatic, listen patiently, then help find a solution.

9. **Provide a Kitchen Calendar for the Homeworker.** See to it that all appointments and plans that involve the homeworker are posted there.

10. **Take Care of Yourself.** Take your breaks away from the client without feelings of guilt. Be realistic about how much you can do before reaching that "burnout" stage.

Section III

The Caregiver or Homeworker: Family/Friend/Family Member/ Professional

It isn't the mountain ahead that wears you out—it's the grain of sand in your shoe.
Robert Service

14

Who Fills the Role of Caregiver or Homeworker?

This section is crammed with information and has a theme: *All you ever wanted to know about being an exceptional homeworker—a caregiver or domestic worker—but didn't know how to ask.*

Like an advocate, a caregiver or a domestic worker can be anyone—a friend, family member, or professional. Formal education is not mandatory; some people just have a knack of knowing how to minister to the needs of others. You do not have to be as strong as Hercules or as compassionately ambitious as Florence Nightingale. Lesser strengths and motivations go a long way in assisting those in need.

In this section, matters pertaining to the homecare worker are the major focus, and you may consider a paid family member or friend as a professional, just as you would a stranger who receives pay for services.

In any case, the information in Section III will be of help to all types of homeworkers who either volunteer or work for pay in a client's home. Family members or friends need not concern themselves with agency relationship and interview presentation.

Both caregivers and domestic workers are homeworkers, but they play different roles and we will look at those now. Keep in mind that the two things that are most important when working in another person's home are common to both types of workers. These two things are (1) that you respect the client and the client's property, and (2) that you deliver the best service possible.

Caregivers and domestic workers may be part-time, full-time, or live-in workers. By Internal Revenue Service definition, these workers can work as independent contractors, self-employed workers, or employees. In Section I, pages 55-56, and in this section under Agency/Homeworker Relationship, pages 140–141, you will find listed the conditions that determine a worker's IRS employment status. The standard roles of domestic workers and caregivers are defined as follows.

Domestic Worker

A domestic worker has responsibility for an area or areas of the client's home. You may be a homemaker, cook, chauffeur, gardener, valet, personal assistant, or maid, or a combination of any of these. You will not be directly responsible for the physical, mental, or emotional well-being of the client, but the manner in which you perform your duties may influence all those things.

As a domestic worker, you will be judged by the thorough and conscientious performance of your domestic duties. If you are a homemaker, you will show your expertise and pride by having on display the neatest, cleanest house on the block. If you are a chauffeur, you will drive the cleanest car, in the most careful fashion, on the most convenient routes to your client's destinations. If you are a gardener, you will look with satisfaction upon neat grounds that you tend with a sensitive and knowing touch.

Not only will you derive immense gratification from the job you have done well, but you will be valued by, and grow in value to, the client for whom you work. The benefit of your thorough and conscientious performance of your job, other than that which meets the eye and is obvious, is the confidence and peace of mind your client reaps from your efforts.

Lilith, age 83

When I hired Delma to help me out, I was doubtful about the entire situation. I had always tended my own affairs and had little confidence that any other person would be efficient enough to suit me.

Much to my relief, Delma was not only efficient, but she was also bright, cheerful, and very energetic. She even took care of my patio plants and the birds.

Delma has worked for me for two years now and I wonder how I ever got along without her.

Caregiver

As a caregiver, you are doing just that: giving care. You may give this care as a companion, a home health aide (HHA), a certified nurse assistant (CNA), a licensed practical nurse (LPN), or as a registered nurse (R.N.). Most companions, HHAs, and CNAs will work as part-time, full-time, or live-in workers. LPNs and R.N.s are more likely to work part time or regular eight-hour or twelve-hour shifts. Also, most caregivers work under the IRS status of "employee" for either a client or an agency. For factors that determine a worker's IRS status, see pages 140–141.

Family members and friends who receive compensation from the client for filling any of the above positions must determine how to handle that income. That many workers in those categories are paid cash and do not declare those cash payments on their tax returns makes the Internal Revenue Service very unhappy. However, it does happen.

For anyone who does not receive a Form 1099 MISC at the end of the year and who does not declare income of this nature, whether or not they do receive a 1099 MISC, there are negative aspects to consider: coping with a guilty conscience, and paying back taxes, penalties, and interest if the Internal Revenue Service catches up with you. For the client, there are also adverse consequences of paying a worker "under the table" and not issuing an IRS W-2 Form or 1099-MISC. The first is that it prevents the client from claiming any portion of those payments as medical expense if those services were rendered as healthcare services. The second is that the client may have to pay a fine and some or all of those back taxes.

Sally, age 27

I got this really great job as a nurse aide doing a twelve-hour night shift. It wasn't really hard because Mr. Elderva slept most of the night.

The thing was, I wanted my pay in cash. I mean, a check would have been all right, I just didn't want taxes taken out or a W-2, or anything. I was going to college to be an R.N., and I needed every cent of my pay. Well, I *was* making $600 a week, but it didn't seem like a regular job.

But when I asked Mr. Elderva to pay me in cash and why, he gave me an earful. After he explained how he could get a break on his taxes because I provided medical help, I saw his point.

From there, I learned about estimated tax payments, Social Security and Medicare withholding, and that darned old form, the 1099-MISC. Oh, well, I just figured it wouldn't hurt to ask.

Most of the time it isn't greed that spurs a worker to cut corners, it is need. However, abiding by IRS guidelines is the best course to take. Regardless of your working status, stay square. Work within legal and valid IRS parameters, and within those parameters, you need to establish a sterling personal background and solid professional credentials.

15

Establishing Personal Background and Professional Credentials

A worker's *background* and *credentials* will be evidenced by personal references, professional references, and professional licenses. You, the worker, can present an impressive professional history by organizing all licenses and references in a concise file. It is this portfolio that will open doors to the most desirable jobs in the home-care field.

Personal background

Part of your background file will be personal references attesting to your good character. These references will be letters from people who have known you the longest. Exclude family members when soliciting these letters and rely only on old friends. Family members are not good candidates for personal references because they would, of course, be suspected of bias.

Zelda, age 65
I always take my file folder with my letters of reference, my résumé, and my nurse's license and certifications with me to every interview. I find

this documentation puts a certain light in a prospective client's eye.

The cost of the folder and copies is negligible, and making them available to a prospective client puts me ahead of the competition. As a matter of fact, I've had several clients tell me that's why they hired me; I left them hard evidence of my experience and good character. They had names to check, telephone numbers to call. They knew I wasn't holding anything back.

If your friends feel awkward writing personal recommendations, assure them that the letters they write will be just fine. These letters do not have to be typewritten. Handwritten letters from old friends vouching for your good character are respected testimonials.

The letters can attest to your sense of duty, your honesty, reliability, sincerity, your sense of humor, stable personality, your patience, your compassion, and your caring nature. If you have friends of ten-, twenty-, or thirty-years' duration, those friends should have no problem finding good qualities about you to endorse.

If the letter writers have no objections, have them place their telephone number at the bottom of the letter. Be sure the letters are dated. Make file copies, as the letters will never be obsolete and can be used for years. What your friends have to say about your basic character should never change.

In addition to personal references from others, you will want to compose a brief personal history. You needn't go into great detail, but do include your birthplace, birth date, home address, and a few of your personal interests and hobbies.

You do not *have* to give this information, of course. But if you were the client, wouldn't you want to know something about the person coming into your home? Give the client enough information so you will not be a total stranger when you first begin employment.

Credentials to establish

The two kinds of credentials you want to establish are professional references and professional licenses.

Professional references are letters from previous clients, the clients' relatives, or the clients' friends that attest to your value as a homeworker. If you have performed your job duties well and left your positions under amiable circumstances, you should have had no trouble leaving with reference letters.

A client may be unable to write a letter on his or her own, or your job may have ended because of a client's death. In either of these cases, ask a relative or friend of the client—one who was familiar with you and your job situation—to write the letter. Do not hesitate to request a letter of reference. The request is a reasonable one, and one that most people will not hesitate to fill.

If you are leaving a client under unfavorable circumstances, even though you may not have caused those circumstances, you must not expect a letter of reference. Do not ask a friend of the client or a member of the client's family to write one either. You would be asking that they compromise their loyalty to the client.

In a case such as this, in your references or on your résumé under "reason for leaving" (a job), just put "to change jobs." If anyone questions that notation, you may explain, if you wish.

Erin, age 42

My listing of references was pretty complete. I had listed all my previous employers and the positions I had held with them. One thing that didn't look just right on my list was how often I had changed jobs. I got questioned a lot about that.

> All I had to do was explain that I came from a resort town where people came and went every few months. That cleared that issue up every time. I finally got smart and just wrote that in the list.

To ensure that you will leave a job with a good professional reference, be diligent and conscientious in performing all duties. Use every ounce of patience and all the professional skills you possess to give exemplary service. You will be building the professional reputation that is your bread and butter, and the better that reputation is, the more bread and butter you will have.

The other kinds of credentials you want to have are professional licenses. Companions and domestic workers—maids, valets, homemakers, gardeners—usually will not have professional licenses. Other workers as listed below *will* have licenses.

- **Chauffeur**: A chauffeur will have a class of driver's license that will authorize him or her to drive for hire.
- **Cook**: A cook will have a certificate or diploma from a school of culinary arts. In most households, nutrition classes and/or professional references will be adequate and will substitute for formal training.
- **Home Health Aide**: A home health aide will have a course completion certificate and certificates for adult CPR, standard first aid, HIV/Aids, and needs continuing education credits to keep HHA certificate active.
- **Certified Nurse Assistant** (may be designated as certified nurse *aide*): A nurse assistant or aide will have a numbered certificate that can be checked for authenticity with the appropriate state agency and certificates for adult CPR, first aid, and HIV/Aids. This type of worker also needs continuing education credits to keep CNA certificate active.

- **Licensed Practical Nurse**: A licensed practical nurse must have a diploma from an accredited school, pass state boards, and have continuing education credits.
- **Registered Nurse**: A registered nurse must have a diploma from an accredited school, pass state boards, and have continuing education credits to keep RN license active.

One other type of professional license is a personal liability bond, sometimes called a fidelity bond, which can be taken out through an insurance company. A bonded worker will find a client more trusting and at ease knowing that the worker comes with "honesty insurance."

The bonding process is simple and inexpensive. You need give only basic personal information and a $25,000 bond can cost as little as $200 a year. The professional homeworker will find that a bond greatly enhances that worker's desirability as an employee.

Whatever you do, you, the worker, must *never* alter or fake a license. Even if you register with an agency and get by with the deception there, the client may decide to verify your license. Do the work necessary to earn your license, then do that which is necessary to keep your license valid and current.

The same goes for the personal identification you give when applying for a job. Never use a false driver's license, green card, birth certificate, or passport. Operating under false identification is not only illegal, but it can also be nerve-wracking for you. Take the time, expend the energy, and spend the money that will keep all your identifying and professional papers in order.

Aieda, age 23

My green card had expired. I didn't know what to do. I needed to work for my family. I am a good worker, I work hard. But my papers gave out.

For money, I got papers, but I worried all the time. People would find out. I would have big trouble. I knew a nurse who had a fake license, she didn't worry. But I did.

At last, I told the people I worked for. I trusted them, they were nice. When they said they would help, I was so happy. Now I work with good papers again. I don't worry.

Once you have all of your personal references, professional references, and professional licenses together, make plenty of copies, and decide the format you will use to present them to agencies and prospective clients.

You can build a neat file by placing your papers in a simple two-pocket file folder. If you have résumé material, but do not know how to put it in résumé form, take it to a typing service (found in the Yellow Pages). A typist there usually can give you a completed résumé and several copies for under thirty dollars.

Having been hired in the past as a homeworker and having had no résumé, you may ask why you need one now. The answer is that you are a professional and you need a professional presentation. And if you register with an agency, you enter into a relationship with other professionals, a relationship that can last a long time and give your professional life added credibility. In all matters pertaining to your job, always look, act and present yourself in a professional manner.

16

The Agency/Homeworker Relationship

Many domestic and healthcare homeworkers prefer to list with agencies. Others prefer to advertise, interview, and be hired on their own.

If you are one of those homeworkers who prefer to use an agency as an employment base, you can do this in several ways . . . through a domestic staffing agency, a homemaker/sitter/companion agency (h/s/c agency), a nurse registry, or through a home healthcare agency. All four types of agencies are involved in the business of matching workers to jobs in private homes, but in most states a domestic staffing agency or an h/s/c agency cannot place healthcare workers because they do not hold certain required state and/or federal licenses.

Domestic staffing agencies specialize in placing domestic (home staff) workers such as cooks, homemakers, maids, valets, chauffeurs, gardeners, and sometimes, nannies and *au pairs*. These agencies take applications from workers and requests (job orders) from prospective clients. After checking references and background information on applicants and then analyzing the needs of clients, the agency sets up an interview between a particular client and the worker(s) best suited to that client's needs.

After the agency has matched a client to a worker and placed the worker in the client's home, the agency waits a stipulated trial period to test the compatibility of the client and the worker. After the trial period, the agency collects from the client a placement or "finder's" fee. The worker should have to pay no fee.

Until a few years ago, there were a number of employment agencies that did charge the worker a fee, sometimes as much as a full month's pay, which the worker could remit in installments. Because a few of these agencies are still in operation, it is important that you, the worker, ask about fees during your initial contact with any agency.

Also, when you register with an agency, ask if the agency offers ongoing support once you have been placed with a client. Many of them do not.

B.J., age 36

Dr. Leon was a nice man. I enjoyed my job as homemaker with him. The only thing was, he was impatient with the workers the agency sent out for him. I learned to cope with his impatience and stayed on the job for a year.

At the end of that year, I asked for a raise of fifty cents an hour. He said yes, but changed his mind a few days later.

I called Winona at the staffing agency and asked if she would please talk to the doctor. She said she would, but just as a friend, not in any official capacity because she usually didn't do that.

She knew just how to talk to him, apparently, because the raise was on my next check—not retroactive, mind you—but I was happy.

A good agency representative will be eager to help, if necessary. More often than not, the representative wants to keep contact with both the client and the worker and provide future placement services for either or both, should the opportunity arise.

As opposed to domestic and staff workers, healthcare workers (caregivers) register and are hired through nurse registries or home healthcare agencies. Listings of the differences between domestic staffing agencies, h/s/c agencies, nurse registries, and healthcare agencies can be found in Section I, pages 54–60.

One primary difference in agencies is the role an agency assumes in the employer/employee relationship. Unlike most other types of agencies, a home healthcare agency usually treats the worker as its direct employee. Most domestic staffing agencies, h/s/c agencies, and nurse registries treat workers as independent contractors *within* the agency and as a direct employee of the client. If you, the worker, are an independent contractor with an agency, payroll arrangements are left up to you and the client who will be your direct employer. It is important for you, the worker, to understand the fine distinctions between being an *independent contractor* and being an *employee*.

An independent contractor is a worker who (1) sets the hours to be worked, (2) determines the duties to be carried out, and (3) supplies the equipment needed to perform those duties. The client can outline the job to be done, but the worker is supposed to have the freedom to determine how the job is done, which tools and equipment to use on the job, and the time within which the job will be completed.

An independent contractor is responsible for keeping tax records and paying all Social Security, Medicare, and income tax payments required by the Internal Revenue Service. In a domestic staffing situation and in many homecare situations, a homeworker is usually placed in a job situation by an agency and then works directly for the client. Treating the worker as an independent contractor relieves the domestic staffing agency, an h/s/c agency, or a nurse registry from employer responsibility for a worker. The worker they place becomes an employee of the client and the client assumes employer responsibility for that worker.

Under *employee* status, a worker performs services that the client dictates, follows a schedule set by the client, and looks to the client to supply all materials and tools essential to the performance of the job. The employee worker is responsible for all income taxes (unless the employer wants to pay them) and half of Social Security and Medicare payments. The client is responsible for the remaining half of Social Security and Medicare payments, federal unemployment tax, and Worker's Compensation (if required).

As a homeworker, decide under which IRS designation you are going to work. Do not wait until April when your taxes are due to decide you want to be an employee instead of an independent contractor. If you do, your client will be miffed, and understandably so. (See Appendix B for sources of more information.)

Adele, age 50

My mother needed a health aide and I found one. But I made a big mistake. I believed the aide when she said she would take care of her own deductions and taxes.

Early in March, the aide said she needed $3,000 to pay her taxes and withholding on the wages Mother had paid to her. I was floored.

After speaking with Mother's accountant and then to an IRS clerk, I learned that the aide was responsible for all of her taxes and half the amounts she owed for Social Security and Medicare. By IRS standards, she was an employee.

The aide said she hadn't realized that. I was skeptical, but gave her the benefit of the doubt, and Mother paid what was right according to the IRS. The aide stayed on, but I had her sign a statement that she agreed to withholding and would pay all her own taxes. From that time on, we let Mother's accountant take care of payroll.

You, the worker, must also be clear about the *type* of worker you are. There are instances in which a home health aide, nurse aide, or a nurse registers with a domestic staffing agency or an h/s/c agency as a companion and is hired in that capacity only to find that on the job they are rendering some form of medical assistance. In a case such as this, the domestic staffing agency cannot be faulted for lacking the required healthcare license(s) and placing someone who renders medical services on the job. The worker entered the position as non-medical personnel. What happens after the date of hire is strictly between the client and the worker. If you, the worker, find yourself in a similar situation, take heed—state and federal regulations require that you have certain training, certifications, and licenses if you are to deliver medical services. If you perform duties for a client that you have not been trained and licensed to perform, you could be opening yourself up to fines and prosecutions.

As stated earlier in this section, you must never give an agency or a client false references or false identifying information. Also, you must be honest with the agency or client, and state outright the kinds of job duties you are, or are not, willing to perform. Be clear about the type of job you want and the schedules you can work.

An agency supervisor cannot read your mind and has no time to play Worker Tic-Tac-Toe, moving you from job to job until, by pure chance, you find the very job you didn't let that supervisor know you wanted in the first place. Nor should a client suffer because of your indecision.

You have a responsibility to give an agency adequate and accurate information that the agency can use to match your best abilities to a client's most important needs. The agency can then set up and send you to interviews that, because of your professionalism, will result in your gainful employment.

To prepare for interviews and to make them productive, you, the worker, will devote a lot of time and serious attention to interview presentation.

17

Interview Presentation

A client's first impression of you, the worker, will be formed at the job interview, and the manner in which you present yourself during this interview is crucial.

Be sure you are on time for the interview—even five minutes early is acceptable. Arrive too early, and you may inconvenience the client.

Make certain that you have understandable directions to the interview location, either from the agency or from the client. If you have time, make a dry run the day before the scheduled interview, so that you know exactly where you are going. If you will be using public transportation, check schedules ahead of time and allow for traffic and weather delays.

When you arrive for the interview, after introductions, present your information portfolio to the client, and tell the client that you welcome questions.

During the interview, observe the client closely. If your duties include lifting or transferring the client, calculate your strength and ability right then.

Be aware of your immediate reactions to the client. Do you feel you will be comfortable working with the client? Do you feel reasonably at ease with the atmosphere in the client's home?

Homeworkers, especially caregivers who work closely with the client, must be discerning when assessing and accepting a job. Working one-on-one with a client in a home setting is always stressful to some degree. Workers who ignore gut instincts when assessing a job are doing themselves *and* the client a grave disservice.

Genevieve, age 32

While I interviewed with Mrs. Lynn, I felt something was wrong, but couldn't put my finger on it. I thought she was tense because of the interview. She was very quiet, but nice, and seemed agreeable to little changes I wanted on the job description—going in at eight in the morning instead of seven, taking my two-hour break at two in the afternoon, instead of at one.

Still feeling uneasy, I took the job as her companion. I soon found she had a negative attitude about everything. She even wanted to renege on the changes we'd agreed on.

She stayed distant and unhappy. I was having some bad times myself, and after a while, I was as unhappy as she was—not very professional, but I couldn't help it.

I should have paid attention to that feeling I had during the interview. I tried, but my own lousy attitude wasn't doing either of us any good, so I quit, and I really think she was glad to see me go.

As the interview progresses, allow the client to talk without interruption and listen intently. After the interviewer has finished speaking, ask questions—questions about the requirements for uniforms, work schedules, and the number of clients involved. Ask for a written job description, and if no written job description is available, ask if the client or you, yourself, can make a list of the specific duties in the position being offered.

Often, a client's job description is vague or incomplete, and soon after beginning a job, you, the worker, may find that you are doing many chores not included in the job description and not mentioned during the interview. The interview is an opportune time to initiate a practice that both the client and the advocate have been advised to use. It is this: Any time you have questions about an issue between you and the client . . .

DISCUSS—DECIDE—PUT IT IN WRITING.

Then both you and the client will sign and date a resolution form like the one found in Section I, page 24.

If you have a written base from which to build, you can discuss and effectively negotiate payroll or duty issues, which come up *after* you are already hired.

Maisie, age 31

When I took a job as a maid I received a very detailed job description. I was glad, because I had trouble on previous jobs when my duties hadn't been set out clearly. All my duties on this job were normal maids' duties.

Three weeks after I started, the housekeeper handed me a leash and told me to walk the dogs, all four of them. That same afternoon, the gentleman I worked for asked me to pick up a grocery order at the market.

I asked him if we could talk. We went over my job description again, then agreed to my two new duties and an additional fifty dollars a week for me to do them.

If the interview goes well and the client considers you a good prospect for hire, you may be shown around the client's house or condo. As you take the tour, ask questions about the position you are applying for. Show sincere interest in the client's surroundings and daily routine. If you are a healthcare worker instead of a companion or domestic worker, you will ask about the client's:

- Sleeping habits
- Eating regime
- Hearing or sight problems
- Special therapies, range of motion, or exercise
- Use of durable equipment (walkers, breathing devices, wheelchairs, etc.)
- Frequency of visits to the doctor(s)
- Special accommodations needed for travel

If you are interviewing for a domestic position, make a list of questions about specific duties. Use your list, along with the client's job description, to define the parameters of the job.

While you are asking questions and assessing the job and the client, the client is also assessing you and may decide to offer you the job at the interview. If this happens, you may have made your own decision and be able to give the client a definite yes or no answer.

If you decide the job is not right for you, politely explain why you are refusing the position: "I appreciate your offer, but I don't feel I can take the job because . . ." and then give the reason: "The schedule doesn't suit me," or "I do not have the physical strength the job requires."

You may have discovered during the interview that there are *clients*, instead of *a client*, and you may give that as your reason for refusing the job. If you need time to consider the offer, ask for no longer than a day or two. The client has needs to be met and cannot be expected to wait an extended period of time.

If you obtained the interview through an agency, the agency will be contacted by the client after the interview, and the agency representative will contact you to discuss your hire status.

Before you accept a job, make sure that you have evaluated that job correctly, and be absolutely certain that it fits your personal employment needs.

18

Evaluating a Job for Your Personal Employment Needs

To make a thorough evaluation of a prospective position, you must consider at least seven distinct aspects of that position: (1) physical work environment, (2) physical condition of the client, (3) transportation to and from the job, (4) work schedules, (5) pay rate, (6) your compatibility with the client, and (7) whether the job is short-term or long-term, temporary or permanent.

When considering these job aspects, be thorough in your consideration and honest about what you need and want from a job.

Physical work environment

How flexible are you about your private space on the job? If you are a live-in worker, is your room too small, too large, or too close to the center of activity in the home? Do cream and beige rob you of energy, are you irritated by green and pink? As amusing as these questions may seem, spending time in surroundings that are not soothing to you is no laughing matter. Because a client will not be seeing your accommodations through your eyes, you will have to bring up the subject of change.

Daisy, age 56

My whole lifetime, I've been sensitive to color. It may have come from having artists for parents.

Anyway, the job I had was a live-in position, and I had a beautiful private bedroom and bath. But the colors were all wrong—brown, beige, dark wood, antiques. I really missed the brighter colors in my bedroom at home.

I got up my nerve, finally, and asked my employer if I could redecorate. She couldn't bring herself to change that part of her home, but she moved me to a different bedroom/bath area. The new room was done in blues and greens and got lots of light. It was a good move. I felt different and more alive, enough so that my employer complimented me on my "better disposition."

Is a condo environment too restrictive for you? Do you prefer the spaciousness of a house with grounds? As in any job, the hours you spend at work should be spent in a setting conducive to a settled state of mind.

Physical condition of the client

Will the position offered require that you lift or transfer the client? Are you confident of your ability to perform those movements? Think weeks and months ahead—do you think you can hold out over the long term?

Is the client bedridden or unable to walk without assistance? Will you be required to sit with the client for long periods each day? Can you do that without becoming bored, impatient, or irritated?

You must never go into a job knowing that you will be impatient or bored with a client. The money you make from the job will not compensate for the drain of mental and emotional energy you will suffer.

Transportation to and from the job

Do you have reliable transportation? If using public transportation, how much time and money will you spend? Will your earnings from the job make up for your transportation time and expense? Is your private or public transportation reliable? Do you have a backup plan if your primary transportation plan fails?

A reliable transportation plan is vital, not only because it is important that you get to and from your job each day, but also because it is important that you are consistently on time, that you impress your client with your punctuality and reliability.

Schedule

Be realistic about a schedule that suits you. Do not compromise this point by taking a job that requires you to work more or fewer hours than you want or need to work.

Avis, age 25

I loved working as a home health aide, but I needed more money. I couldn't find another shift to fit in with the one I already had, so I took a second job knowing I would have to report only an hour after I got off the first job.

My big mistake was forgetting how long it would take to get across town from one job to the other.

I began leaving my first job a few minutes earlier (and earlier, and earlier), until that client got upset enough to tell me I couldn't leave early anymore. Then I kept being late for my evening job, and that client was so nice, but he needed his evening meal and meds right on time, so my being late messed up his schedule.

I had to face it. I couldn't keep both jobs. I quit the evening job, which I hated doing because that

client was a gem. But I learned the hard way that
I had to be honest about my physical limitations.

If you need to earn more money, you can work two
jobs, of course, but you may run into scheduling and
transportation problems. If you need or want fewer hours
than a job offers, you must keep searching for another
job. Never take a job with a view to "cutting down" on
your hours later, thus inconveniencing a client.

Pay Rate

The issue of what is or is not adequate pay for a particular job can be especially difficult to work out. Ballpark
figures for different types of workers are given in Section I, page 59. Unless you work for a home healthcare
agency that charges the client and then pays you, you
will have a major say about the rate of pay you receive
for your services.

Homeworkers who hire out through some types of
agencies determine for themselves which pay rates are
acceptable. During the interview and from the job description, you will assess a job and decide upon a range
of pay acceptable to you. You and the client can then . . .

DISCUSS—DECIDE—PUT IT IN WRITING.

When considering a job that involves an inordinate
amount of time, attention, and/or skill, you will want to
request a higher rate of pay, or at least note on the job
description a provision for an increase in pay after you
have proven your abilities on the job. Give the client
three to six months to appreciate your professionalism
and then have the increase go into effect.

You also want to have in the job description provi-
sions to cover changes in the client's general health. Such
changes can cause a job to become more time and labor

intensive, and a worker's pay rate should change accordingly.

Bottom line: Never accept a job without certain knowledge of your pay rate and your pay schedule.

Compatibility with the client

Your compatibility with a new client will not be in question for long. After a week or two, a month at most, you will know if you and the client have conflicts serious enough to preclude a harmonious working relationship. Often in an abrasive relationship, the reason for conflict cannot be isolated. The strain is "just there."

Do not remain in a position where you and the client are incompatible. If you are unhappy on your job, your presence there will be detrimental, not only to you, but also to your client.

Temporary or permanent, short-term or long-term employment

You know how long you want to work; your prospective client does not. If you want *temporary* or short-term employment, do not take a permanent or long-term position with quitting in mind.

If you are looking for a *permanent* or long-term position, you might be tempted to take a temporary or short-term position until you find the job you want. However, this would be unfair to a client, as you would quit and leave that client without a worker.

If you define a prospective job by looking at the seven aspects above, you will place yourself in a good position to exercise your domestic or homecare skills to the fullest. And to help you do that, you need to consider arrangements for your on-the-job needs and, if applicable, live-in arrangements.

19

On-the-Job Needs/Live-In Arrangements

On-the-job needs are much the same for both a live-in worker and a shift worker. Living-in arrangements are of concern only to the live-in worker. And a friend or family member who works in either capacity will face the same issues in these areas that a professional worker will face.

Since the client/homeworker relationship is unique, both on-the-job needs and live-in arrangements should be thoroughly . . .

DISCUSSED—DECIDED—PUT IN WRITING

. . . by the client and the worker *before* a job begins.

Because the client's home is a more personal setting than an office, a sales floor, or an assembly line, a homeworker must give careful consideration to having on-the-job needs met. Doing so necessitates that you, the worker, confront and settle issues that most workers never face.

These issues include social interaction with the client's friends and family members, responsibility for the client's personal property, use of the worker's automobile for the client's convenience, and the interaction the worker has with the client on a personal level.

Three practical matters you will consider are parking rules, work schedules, and arrangements for receiving mail. You will face other more subjective issues: telephone use, on job visits by friends and family members, relationships with other homeworkers, and—especially for the live-in worker—private time and sleeping arrangements.

Before you accept a job, make sure you have examined all of these relevant issues. While examining each issue from your viewpoint, remember to pause occasionally and try to see it from the client's perspective, as well.

Socializing with the Client's Friends and Family Members.

No matter how at ease you may feel in the client's home and around the client's circle of friends and family, you are still a worker in the household. Be friendly and cordial to everyone associated with the client, but never assume that you will be included in any visit, outing, or conversation that the client has with friends or family members.

Miranda, age 39

When I interviewed with Mrs. Green, she talked a lot about going out for lunch and dinner at her favorite restaurants. She also talked about being lonely and needing company.

I had been working as her companion for less than a week when she announced she would be going out for lunch the next day.

The next day I dressed in suitable attire for a visit to Estrella's, the restaurant she had mentioned, and joined her in the sitting room at eleven-thirty. She looked taken aback, and after an awkward pause, told me she would be meeting a friend for a private lunch.

I didn't take my *un*invitation as a personal affront. I took it as a simple misunderstanding on my part. After that, I made a point of asking specifically if she wanted my company.

When the client has a scheduled social function or a friend or family visit, ask the client if your presence is desired or necessary. If a visitor "pops in" on the client, ask if you are needed, and if not, ask the client to let you know if or when you are needed, then excuse yourself.

Responsibility for the Client's Property

As a homeworker, you are in a unique position of responsibility. Unlike a factory, store, or office worker who is responsible for business property only, you are responsible for a work environment that includes the personal property of the client. Your honesty and integrity need to be unquestioned.

Because there will be other people in and out of the client's home constantly—other workers, friends, family members, perhaps casual acquaintances—you, the worker, need to be aware of the placement of the client's personal belongings. Although it is best *not* to know safe combinations and the locations of the client's most valuable possessions such as jewelry, you want to make note of valuable artwork and collectibles—not that you want to serve as household security, but you want to know what is what and that items remain in their usual places.

Jordan, age 42

I have been employed in many households, both as houseman and valet. After working several jobs where some of my clients' valuables went missing, I became extremely paranoid.

In my present job, houseman for a well-known businessman, I rather overstepped my bounds by photographing every precious item in the house.

> I was just finishing up a fourth pack of Polaroid when my employer walked in. When I explained what I was doing and why, he looked amused and said he already had in his possession a detailed inventory.
>
> I was almost embarrassed, but not quite, and told him I would like to keep the photographs on file in case I should notice anything amiss. He agreed, and I must say, I do feel better about it all.

There are, unfortunately, those homeworkers who are not honest. Thefts do take place. If a theft should occur in your place of employment, be ready and willing to take a polygraph test. If a test is requested, do not take the request as a personal affront. This is an ideal moment to put yourself in the client's shoes. What would you want done if a cherished item disappeared from *your* home?

Use of Your Personal Vehicle on the Job

This issue can become a source of extreme conflict if you neglect to have a clear understanding with the client at the inception of your working relationship.

Here are several points pertaining to the use of vehicles on the job for you, as a homeworker, to consider:

1. Never use your car to transport a client or the friends and family members of the client without a *waiver of responsibility*. Consult your auto insurance agent and/or a lawyer, and let that expert tell you what to do to be within the law when using your vehicle to transport others.

2. If you are placed by a healthcare agency, the agency will provide you with set rules governing car use.

3. If you use your vehicle for the client's benefit, you will be providing an additional service to the client. You will be within your rights to request that the client pay a

weekly or monthly stipend to help with insurance, gas, upkeep, and depreciation for your vehicle.

4. If you have use of the client's vehicle, the client assumes the greater responsibility and risk, but you must use the utmost care and respect when in possession of that vehicle. Never drive it without the client's permission, and abstain from using it for your personal business.

5. If you are a chauffeur, or a driver for hire, be certain that you have a contract outlining all the duties and liabilities that you have in that capacity.

Your Interpersonal Relationship with the Client

Intimacy with the client should come slowly, with time. Do not rush a client with informalities. Do not enter gushing, "We're going to be just the best friends," or "I know I'm going to feel just like family here," or "Oh, you remind me so much of my own dear mother." You get the picture—gushing is not professional.

Keep a respectful emotional and physical distance from the client until you have been on the job long enough, usually a year or longer, to truly know the client. Even then, allow the client to set the boundaries of the relationship that the two of you develop.

A "too chummy" relationship can be annoying and uncomfortable for the client, and perhaps for you as well. The client may become interested in your personal life to the extent that you have no privacy on the job.

On the other hand, if you become too involved in the client's personal life, you will be imposing and possibly cause the client to resent even the slightest familiarity on your part. So, even though the client may open the door for immediate interaction with you on a more personal basis, use restraint until you have had time to assess your job and everyone connected with it.

Parking

Wherever you work, a condo, apartment, or a private home, you will find there are specific rules for parking. Observe those rules. Do not cause the client embarrassment or inconvenience by parking in an area other than that designated for you.

If a neighbor of the client challenges your right to park in a certain space, do not argue. Move your vehicle to a neutral area, then inform the client and let the client and the neighbor settle the issue.

Work schedule

The schedule you work will have been agreed upon and acknowledged in writing by you and the client during your interview or by the beginning of your first day of work. Follow that work schedule strictly. Your job affords you no extra flexibility just because you perform your duties in a home setting.

You will instill trust and confidence in the client by arriving at work promptly, taking rest and meal breaks as agreed upon, and by working through the very last minute of your scheduled work day.

Never shirk duties or manipulate the time you spend actually doing work for the client. In other words, don't be on the telephone or working a word puzzle if you are supposed to be cooking or doing laundry.

At the time you accept a job, you need to be honest and realistic about the hours and the days you can and will work. For example, if you take a job knowing that Sunday hours are required, do not use "going to church" as an excuse at a later date to avoid working on Sunday.

Make the client aware at the outset of a job which hours and days that you absolutely will not or cannot work.

Receiving Mail

If you work daily shifts, you have no reason to receive mail at the client's address. Avoid having mail delivered at your work address, even packages from UPS. If you cannot be at home when you expect deliveries, make arrangements with your friends or family members to receive deliveries for you.

Even if you are working a live-in job, always receive mail at your own address. If you have no private residence, rent a post office box near your workplace. A client knows that you must receive mail and will arrange time for you to leave the job to pick it up.

If you insist on receiving mail at the client's address, you are asking for complications in three ways.

1. Your mail may be misplaced with the mail of the client.

2. The client's mail may be misplaced with your mail.

3. When your job with the client ends and you fill out and file a "change of address" card at the post office, errors can occur. First-class mail addressed to you may continue to be delivered to the client's address and/or first-class mail addressed to the client may be delivered to your new address.

Be smart. Keep your mail delivery separate from the client's at all times.

Food and Meals

Guidelines concerning food and meals on the job vary, depending upon whether you are a live-in or shift worker.

A shift worker will usually bring to the job food for snacks and meals. If food requires refrigeration, the worker labels it and stores it in a designated area in the refrigerator. Food stored in a cupboard will be labeled and set aside, as well.

One of the optional considerations a client can make for a live-in worker is the provision of all regular meals at home and payment for meals when the worker accompanies the client to restaurants. Not paid for by the client are a worker's special snacks, diet foods, and excessive amounts of any item—soda, for example. You, the worker, should treat a client's stock of food and drinks with the same respect as you treat all personal property of the client. Most clients want to share and will share freely, but you must always ask if you have the slightest doubt about this matter.

Telephone Use

Every homeworker needs to keep in contact with friends and family members; however, use of the client's private telephone for this purpose can generate tension and resentment on both sides.

On a full-time job that is going to be long-term, you will be well advised to pay for the installation and maintenance of a second line. The client may pay the installation fee, but you should not expect or assume they will.

Phyllis, age 48

Ten years ago, I started working personal homecare as a nurse aide, and I learned fast it wasn't a good idea to use the house phone. On that job, I was on the phone to my daughter when my employer's husband tried to get through with news of a death in the family. I have paid for a phone of my own on all my jobs since then.

On my last job I wanted to put in a phone right away, but Mr. Witt said no. A few days later, I received a call from a friend in Alaska. Only a minute into the call, Mr. Witt picked up the extension phone, then quickly put it down. A minute later, he picked up again.

Then he picked up again. I hurriedly told my friend I would call her from home, then I went into the den and told Mr. Witt he could make his call.

He said, "What call? I don't need to make a call." I was just a little perturbed.

We talked the next morning, and I had a private line hooked up immediately. I got the bill and Mr. Witt and I didn't have to worry about bumping heads on his telephone.

You may have a pager (a beeper) and when paged, be expected by your callers to get in touch immediately. This can pose a problem, because, excluding breaks and meals, you are always on the job. You, being a good homeworker, will make clear to all personal contacts that you can return calls only during rest or meal breaks. Emergencies are, of course, exceptions.

A live-in worker definitely needs a cellular phone or a private line. A schedule of three to seven days and/or nights away from friends and family members is a sure setup for extreme stress and burnout. That you, the worker, have a way to speak in privacy with friends and family members is vital.

On-the-Job Visits by Friends and Family Members

Remember, the informal home setting of your job is no excuse to make your activities on the job informal. Just think, if you were a client, would you want strangers knocking at your door and coming into your home?

Exclude all visits by your personal contacts, or, with the client's knowledge and permission, allow only limited visits. Even if your full attention is not required by the client, you must still be alert and ready to help at all times.

Private Time for the Worker

Private time is more of an issue for the homeworker who lives in than it is for a homeworker who works an eight-, ten-, or twelve-hour shift. A domestic homeworker need not be overly concerned with private time, because a domestic worker usually works away from the client. Contact with the client is not as constant as it is for a companion or a healthcare worker.

A live-in worker, however, needs periods throughout the workday to be alone, sometimes to shake the cobwebs out, and other times to readjust their attitude.

If you are a worker living in the client's home among the client's possessions, despite the fact that the home and possessions may be quite lovely, your personal tastes usually are not reflected in them. This is one of the primary reasons that a live-in arrangement can be stressful for a worker.

If you are a live-in worker, you can only hope that the client understands your special need for more frequent, private relaxation breaks.

Gertie, age 33

The agency I work with places me in all kinds of jobs, some shift jobs, some live-ins. I never have a problem working shifts. I go home and relax. But live-in work is different. It's almost like being married to someone.

I found out quick that on live-in jobs I need a break from my clients every day, and my agency makes sure that my clients know that. I'm not sure they understand that, if I didn't have a break, I'd be too grouchy to put up with.

As it is, I come off my break with a second wind, more patience, and I know I can make it right on through the rest of the day.

Interaction with Other Homeworkers

As much as it is within your power, you have a responsibility to help provide and maintain a tranquil environment for the client. This means that, aside from working well with the client, you will also work well with other homeworkers.

You will, upon occasion, find a co-worker unlikeable, even insufferable. In a worst case scenario, if that worker continues in the employ of the client, you may have to give notice and move on. More often, however, a workable, professional relationship with a difficult co-worker can be established.

A healthcare agency supervisor will help with problems or address the issue of incompatibility between workers employed by the agency and keep the client in a protected, neutral position, if possible.

If you are an independent worker, take the initiative yourself. The first step you take to establish a compatible relationship with a troublesome co-worker is to put yourself in the other worker's shoes, maybe even in the other worker's head. Try to determine the source of the tension between the two of you. Can you talk it out?

Do either of you disapprove of the other's treatment of the client or of the other's job performance?

Do you notice shirking or laziness on the part of the co-worker? Are you shouldering chores that are not legitimately yours? If this is the case, by all means talk to the co-worker, don't tattle to the client.

If a co-worker is uncooperative, unappreciative, and/or uncaring, just back off, stay professional, and do your job as effectively and efficiently as you can. Most clients will spot dissension among or between workers, determine its source, and handle the situation without a worker ever having to bring it up.

Is your relief worker always or often late, making you late for appointments and eroding your time off? If so, you may want to request a meeting with you, the other homeworker, and the client. At this meeting, approach the issue in a mature fashion and be clear when stating your complaint. Be as flexible as you can be in *all* matters, and help your co-workers whenever you can.

Ilana, age 45

Shantal, the nurse who worked weekends, wasn't very friendly and I didn't mind. But we shared the extra bedroom and she left her sheets on the bed and a mess in the bathroom. Every Saturday I had to wash her dirty linens.

Ms. Edwards had health problems and I wasn't going to bother her. After a month of messes I talked to Shantal about it.

She agreed that I left clean sheets and a spotless bathroom for her. She was a bit vacant during our discussion, but finally understood that I wanted her to leave things neat and clean.

We never did get real close, but we got that straight.

Considering the client's best interests, as well as your co-worker's, you should treat all co-workers with respect and consideration, thus creating pleasant working relationships and a calm working environment.

You may be lucky enough to work with a tag-team partner. This is a person with whom you have worked before and know well. You and your tag-team partner will be familiar with each other's personalities, work habits, and personal foibles. You will already have tested your tolerance of each other and know that you are compatible. A tag-team arrangement is advantageous to everyone involved in a homecare situation.

Private Space and Live-in Arrangements

A homeworker, either shift or live-in, should have a quiet place designated for rest and break periods. The worker needs to have an understanding with the client about this and make note of it on the job description.

Live-in workers have designated living quarters and use those quarters for rest breaks, unless the client has agreed that another area of the home—the kitchen, sitting room, or patio is to be used for this purpose.

For sleeping and off-duty time, a live-in worker will usually have a private bedroom and private bath. In a very few households, a worker may be afforded a guest apartment or a guest house.

Most often, private quarters are decorated according to the client's tastes and furnished with the client's personal belongings. If you, the worker, find the decor of your quarters unsettling, discuss with the client changes you might like to make. Be polite, tactful, and sensitive, and never make changes without the client's full knowledge and consent.

20

Money Matters

Money and related matters can be touchy topics, indeed. If you, the worker, are hired through a home healthcare agency, you will have a wage amount, a payroll plan, and benefits determined for you by that agency.

An independent homeworker must consider not only a fair wage for the regular schedule, but also several other issues and money concerns: vacations, paid personal and sick days, raises, reimbursements for monies spent on behalf of the client, bonuses, gifts of any nature, telephone expenses, car expenses, and the handling of the client's finances.

A worker's car and telephone expenses were covered on pages 157 and 161. Now look at these seven other money matters.

1. **Wages**. You know, or should know, what the going pay rate in your area is for the type of work you do. Be fair with yourself, as well as with the client, and do not sulk after a job begins about a pay rate that you agreed upon at the outset of the job.

2. **Raises**. Verify your starting rate of pay during your initial interview with the client. While discussing that pay rate, inquire about raises—how often, how much? As in any job, you and the client need to have

an understanding about raises. You, the worker, want to know what to expect for a job well done and when to expect it. A raise is an incentive and a reward for performance of job duties over and beyond the expectations of the client.

3. **Bonuses.** A bonus is to be *expected* by a worker only once a year and that is at Christmas. A worker is not due a bonus on other holidays or on birthdays. Bonuses that you receive other than the Christmas bonus are optional, to be decided by the client. They are "wheel" bonuses. (Term derived from workers acknowledging that they are working for a generous, understanding client—the worker is "on the wheel," going places.) Even if legitimately deserved, wheel bonuses should be greatly appreciated by all workers who receive them.

4. **Vacations and Paid Days Off.** Again, during your initial interview, both paid and unpaid vacation periods and sick days should have been decided. A vacation taken by the worker during the first twelve months of employment with a client should be taken at the *worker's* expense. After twelve consecutive months of employment with the same client, a one-week paid vacation for the worker is standard, and after two years, a two-week paid vacation is in order. If the client does not agree with these guidelines, you, the worker, may offer alternatives: one week with only one-half week paid, or two weeks with only one week paid.

Periodic time off is a must for a homecare worker, especially a worker who is giving one-on-one healthcare. If the job is physically and/or emotionally demanding, you, the worker, may want to take a week off every three or four months. The client may consider a break every three or four months unreasonable, but explain to the client that these breaks will be beneficial to both of you. A breath of fresh air, some time apart, gives both parties a rest and a chance to objectively evaluate the working relationship. Inevitably, the working relationship resumes after a week's break with both the worker and the client more appreciative of each other, relieved to resume their familiar routine.

5. **Severance Pay.** The worker is owed severance pay in only two situations. The first is when the worker's job ends due to a change in the care plan of the client (needs more advanced care such as an R.N. or moves to an institutional facility), or the job ends because of the client's death. In both of these situations, the job ends because of circumstances that the worker does not cause, and the worker is due at least two week's severance pay—more if the client or the client's family decides so. A worker who quits a job or one who is terminated for unsatisfactory job performance should expect nothing except a last earned paycheck.

Mr. Edgar, age 72

Maxine had been with me three years, and I guess things—you know—changes in her duties and whatnot, just snuck by me. I had hired Maxine to cook, clean, and run errands. Then my niece came to live with me and cooked and cleaned for her rent.

I figured Maxine could wash the car and maybe clean a few windows. She didn't want to.

We tried hashing it out, but then, without warning, Maxine left. Later, she called and wanted vacation pay and two weeks' regular pay. I just sent her pay for the last week she worked. My lawyer said she didn't give me notice and what I sent her was all right.

Unfortunate, the whole thing was. Maxine was a good worker.

6. **Gifts**. You, the worker, will do well to refuse gifts offered by the client, especially those offered during your first year on the job. Be tactful and explain to

the client your policy about gifts. Ideally, your explanation would be given during the initial interview, thus eliminating awkward situations in the future when gifts might be offered. Should you decide to accept gifts, be aware that even a well-meaning client may subconsciously count gifts as additional wages, as a substitute for raises, or as a substitute for a Christmas bonus.

There is also the possibility that you may receive gift items such as clothing, jewelry, or a collectible like a music box that has sentimental value to a member of the client's family. Your acceptance and possession of that item might cause hard feelings, even legal entanglements, at a later date. If you receive such a gift from a client, discreetly consult with a close family member to make certain that the gift was an appropriate one. If the client is afflicted with Alzheimer's or any form of dementia, or if the client is lonely or aging, the act of verifying the validity of a gift becomes even more important. Never take advantage of a client's vulnerability or generous nature.

Della, age 26

I don't know why Mrs. Carl took to me so. We got along, but all I did was my job. After Mr. Carl died, she was sort of lost and I kept her company. I even worked some unpaid hours. I took my job of being a companion very seriously.

Mrs. Carl started giving me jewelry—small, inexpensive things. Then she gave me a stationary box. But then she offered me a diamond watch. I could tell it was expensive. I was concerned about how all this would look to other people, but I hated to hurt her feelings by saying no.

Not long after that, Mrs. Carl insisted that I have one of her Lalique figurines. That did it. I called her daughter. She came the next day and had a long talk with her mother. Mrs. Carl took the watch back. The daughter and I agreed if Mrs. Carl offered me *anything* I was to let her know, and we worked things out like that. I will tell you that some time later the daughter thanked me for being so good to her mother and gave me a bonus.

If you are offered a gift of money, be careful and conscientious if you accept that gift. Again, alert a trusted member of the client's family. This is one instance in which you can break confidence with the client and still be doing the right thing. You may well be protecting the client from him or herself and, in the long run, you can only gain, if not in money, then in self-respect.

7. **Client's Accounts, Credit Cards, and Checkbooks.** If a homeworker is asked to oversee the client's credit cards, checkbooks, or investment accounts, there is only one wise and sensible response: the homeworker should refuse this type of responsibility. If the client is incapable of or does not want to handle financial affairs, the responsibility should be assumed by a friend or family member of the client or by a professional—a lawyer or an accountant.

As a domestic worker, a companion, or a healthcare worker, you are not hired to conduct financial business for the client. If you do involve yourself in the client's financial affairs and questions should arise about the status of those finances, you may find yourself in suspicious circumstances, trying to answer some hard questions. You, the worker, can never be too scrupulous in your handling of any of the client's money. If you purchase items for the client with a credit card or buy groceries for cash, give the client receipts. If the client does not have a receipt file or provide one for you to keep, label an envelope or file folder and maintain a file for the client. Also communicate to the client's advocate or some family member of the client that a receipt file is being kept.

While reading through Money Matters, you may have thought them strongly worded. They are not.

Your professional reputation is built in large part on your honesty and integrity. A professional recommendation will be difficult to elicit from a client who doubts these qualities in you.

As you did with the issues of on-the-job needs, go back now and read again the discussion of the seven issues in Money Matters. Make a list, noting what you expect in the way of wages, raises, vacation periods, etc. Have these figures and facts firmly in mind and down on paper when you interview and *before* you begin a new job. And always be sure that you . . .

DISCUSS—DECIDE—PUT IT IN WRITING.

21

Six Star Tips for Giving Care

Most of the following tips pertain to all homeworkers. Some are more relevant to the companion and the health-care worker. These six-star tips for giving care, if taken seriously, will result in a job performed efficiently in a sensitive, caring manner. The six tips that will enable you to give excellent care are to (1) Understand, (2) Respect, (3) Anticipate, (4) Vent, (5) Inquire, and (6) Detach. Forming an anagram from these words, you will get U R AVID. Avid means eager, and you must be eager in your job to be a good homeworker.

To understand the client, from time to time step into the client's shoes, and imagine how it must feel to have a person, often a stranger, take over personal and household activities–activities that the client was able, at one time, to handle without a second thought.

Understand how difficult it must be for the client to relinquish responsibilities, sometimes major portions of their normal activities—of checkbooks, simple telephone business, driving, or matters of personal hygiene.

Imagine yourself in the client's exact circumstances. And, please, give this imagining more than a fleeting moment. Go to a quiet place, close your eyes, and concentrate. Put yourself, as much as possible, inside the client's world. Stretch your senses. When you do this, you may feel sadly uncomfortable, but you will come close to understanding the client and your job in a way that will be of great benefit to you.

Only with time will you gain the deeper understanding of the client that you need, and over time you may also gain disproportionate feelings of power. These feelings of power grow as you take on more responsibility and exercise more control over the client's daily regime. As this process continues, you come to feel more powerful—the client may feel less so.

This subtle shift of power and control can bring about a condition called Boss Reversal Syndrome. You, the worker, will know if you are afflicted with this syndrome after you answer honestly these questions :

1. Do I feel superior to the client ?
2. Do I get impatient if the client doesn't do what I think the client should do?
3. Am I giving the client commands, instead of suggestions?
4. Am I telling the client what I will and will not do, instead of following my job description?
5. Do I resent the client's comments about my job performance and respond too harshly?

If you answered yes to any of the above questions, reassess your priorities, and remember who is writing your check. The person writing that check is the boss. Within any professional setting there should be no reason to . . .

DISCUSS—DECIDE OR PUT ANYTHING IN
WRITING . . . about this matter.

Respect for all persons is a quality that every home-worker should possess. A homeworker can develop respect for a client by making conscious efforts to understand and empathize with the client.

Domestic homeworkers do not have as much personal contact with clients as companions and healthcare workers have. Still, domestic workers have in their care the client's most treasured possessions. Even a chauffeur will respect and hold the client's well-being and property above all else. A good chauffeur will treat the vehicle(s) in his care with respect and drive in accordance with a client's reasonable and lawful instructions.

Martina, age 55

I went to work for Mrs. Randall after she and her husband divorced.

When we went out, I drove, but she drove me crazy about blowing the horn. Every time we came to an intersection, she would yell, "Blow the horn!"

One day, after about the tenth time she yelled, I just pulled over to the curb and said as calmly as I could, "Mrs. Randall, I only blow a car horn in case of emergency. But this is your car, and it's your horn, so whenever you want the horn to blow, just reach over here and blow it. OK.?"

I was polite when I said it and Mrs. Randall didn't seem to mind that I had said it, and from then on, she didn't yell about that horn anymore.

A homemaker, maid, or cook will knowledgeable about how a client wants the house presented, clothes maintained, and food cooked and served and deliver those services in a diligent manner. When performing duties as directed by a client, you and other homeworkers are not being subservient, you are being professional.

A respectful companion or caregiver will never interject personal beliefs and opinions into the daily activities of the client. As a respectful worker, you will administer care and services in a professional manner, without advocating your own political, religious, or moral agendas. By acting in this manner, you demonstrate to the client the respect you want in return. Keep in mind the Boss Reversal Syndrome and do not fall victim to it.

Anticipate a client's needs by being thoroughly familiar with a client's routine. Your professional services will be invaluable if you can anticipate plan changes and incidental problems.

If a day looms during which the client has a doctor's appointment, a hair appointment, *and* a luncheon appointment, think ahead for both the client and yourself. In your mind, travel through the upcoming day and allow for traffic problems and physical complications. If the client is handicapped and uses special equipment—a wheelchair, an oxygen tank, a walker—allow for "handling" time in and out of stores, offices, and the car.

Lissa, age 45

When I started working as an LPN ten years ago, I wasn't very organized.

My first client, Mr. Hodges, used a wheelchair and wore a hearing aid during the day, and he had a nap every day at two o'clock sharp.

The second week with Mr. Hodges, I had to make an appointment with his psychoanalyst. Without thinking, I booked him a two-thirty appointment. Knowing he would miss his nap threw Mr. Hodges out of sorts, but we went anyway.

In the elevator at the doctor's office, I realized Mr. Hodges didn't have his hearing aid in and we didn't have time to go back and get it. We went on up, but after several minutes of "Huh? Huh?" the doctor set another appointment for Mr. Hodges, and we left his office.

By this time it was raining buckets, and I discovered I hadn't put the umbrella in the wheelchair pocket. After twenty minutes, Mr. Hodges asked me to find a trash bag or something to put over his head, so we could get to the car. He was a very unhappy man.

I had let Mr. Hodges down, and I was devastated. You can believe that whenever we left the house after that I had a checklist, and I was ready for anything.

If the client is facing a serious medical procedure, a family crisis, or an important social function, anticipate the client's emotional state. Stay calm and be prepared to give encouragement and reassurance as needed.

The time and effort you spend to pre-plan daily activities will not only aid the client, but will also make the day less tiring and frustrating for you.

Vent. Please do. If you do not, you will build tension within your workplace and, sooner or later, both you and the client will suffer the effects of that tension.

Why will you be tense? What can cause you frustration? Why would you have to vent? The answer to each of these questions: your constant personal contact with the client. This constant contact fosters the building of tension, resentment, and frustration. Even in the best of circumstances, the client/homeworker relationship can become extremely intense.

In some cases, workers can suffer "nerve damage" from a client's arrogant demeanor, unwarranted criticism, or demands for more or different services. For the worker to react to these things in a petulant or belligerent manner is of benefit to no one. If the worker is respectful and wise, the reaction from that worker will be to say to the client, "I understand your point; may I explain mine to you?" If the situation is downright explosive, the worker will say nothing. Quiet time and reflection will result in a reasonable exchange with the client at some other time. But what to do until then?

As strange as you may think these suggestions to be, try them: Go to a private area where you can speak out loud, and say whatever you wish to say in the tone that suits your mood. Hear yourself say it. Throw a pillow. Stamp your feet (quietly). Have a private, free-for-all venting session and hope that the client is doing the same.

Nathan, age 39

I work as a cook and I'm very impressed with my present employer, Mr. Fitzgerald Haynes-Hiatt, but last weekend I ran into a problem with his attitude—and mine.

Mr. Haynes-Hiatt wanted me to serve a fancy entrée to his guests, and I was up to my apron bib in paté, beef, and filo dough all afternoon.

Mr. Haynes-Hiatt kept calling to the kitchen with changes: "change the dressing. . .change from creamed to mashed . . . yeast rolls to twists. . . ."

I was keeping my patience, flipping the menu this way and that, when in comes Mr. Haynes-Hiatt, himself. He took one look at the entrée and grew red in the face. "I said 'beef, well done,' not *Beef Wellington!*"

Too late. Beef Wellington was served for dinner, while I stood in the soundproof food cooler and ranted at the top of my lungs. After ten minutes of "cooling off," I felt much better.

I did no harm to my reputation or working relationship with Mr. Haynes-Hiatt and later, he actually complimented me on the dinner.

When the time to discuss matters does arrive, you will have dissipated much of your hostility and resentment; only trickles will remain. You will be able to speak in a reasonable and intelligent manner to the client, and you will have avoided causing irreparable damage to your working relationship.

If you don't want to use the methods of venting given above, develop a method that works for you and use it often. You will profit, as will the client, by maintaining a work environment devoid of unnecessary strain.

Inquire about the client's extracurricular interests. Develop curiosity and show interest in the less serious activities in the client's day-to-day routine. In some cases, you will be the only person to show this type of interest.

If the client enjoys watching "Wheel of Fortune," "Jeopardy," or "Kids Say the Darndest Things," watch them with the client. If tennis is the client's greatest passion, even though you haven't the slightest interest in the sport, make an effort and show interest. Allow the client to share with you.

A worker who inquires about the client's hobbies and pastimes gives the client an ego boost and gains knowledge at the same time. If you are curious and inquire, you will gain insight about the client, and you will learn and store information that will serve you well in future job or life situations.

Detach. After all you have read in this section about getting involved with the client, you now need to think about how to detach within the client/worker relationship. You, the worker, want to establish a professional distance between you and the client, so that you can stay objective about the duties you perform. This does not keep you from taking an interest in the client, but it does prevent emotions from running too high in times of stress—either those of the client or your own.

At the very outset of a new job, make a conscious effort to set that professional distance between you and the client. Regardless of how close to the client you may feel or come to feel, your life is still yours and the client's life still belongs to the client. The client comes with personal history of which you have no knowledge, and the client is involved with people of whom you will never be aware. To attempt to become a "best buddy" or confidant is not a wise thing to do. A too-close relationship can result in personal feelings becoming entangled with professional responsibilities and a worker's on-the-job performance suffers. And when a worker's job performance suffers, so does the client. As impossible as you, the worker, may think it to be, you *can* be *involved at a distance*. Take heed, and do just that.

Ten Best Tips
for the Caregiver/Homeworker

1. **Allow the Client To Have Control.** As long as the client is physically safe and taking medications as prescribed, try not to meddle in that client's everyday affairs. Keep your personal opinions about the client's personal life to yourself.

2. **Do Not Fall Victim to the Boss-Reversal Syndrome**. This tip is strongly related to the previous tip and it means just what it says. The client is your boss, you are not the client's boss. For various reasons, you may feel superior to the person for whom you work, but on the job—squelch it.

3. **Respect the Client's History.** Do not meddle in established personal and financial business or in longtime friend and family relationships. As a homeworker, you are hired to give care and support to the client, not to give advice to the client about personal matters.

4. **Slow Down/Speed Up.** Pace your activity and movement to that of the client. Older clients tend to move more slowly and to think in a more deliberate fashion. Be patient. Other clients may move at speeds unthinkable even for the very young and you will have to speed up. Again, be patient.

5. **Take an Interest in the Client's Recreational Activities.** This helps to boost ego and fosters positive self-image in the client. It is not meddling.

6. **Anticipate.** Think through every day before you start through it. Attempt to foresee problems and be ready with solutions.

7. **Do Not Rearrange Items in the Client's Surroundings Without the Client's Request or Permission.** Placing items where you think they are

handiest may seem like a good idea to you. The client, however, may be dismayed and disoriented to find favorite items in unfamiliar places.

8. **Compile Your Own List of Job-related Names, Addresses, and Telephone Numbers.** Because a client may be forgetful or disorganized, you need at your fingertips contact numbers for the client's friends, family members, and doctors. Having the numbers of barbers, grocers, and favorite restaurants comes in handy, also.

9. **Keep Your Personal Possessions Out of the Way on the Job.** Do not leave your purse, books, cell phone, food and drinks, sweaters, sunglasses, car keys, or travel case laying about. Ask the client to designate a space for you to keep personal items that you carry to the job.

10. **Make Every Possible Effort to Work Well with the Client, the Client's Advocate, and Other Homeworkers.** Always walk for a while in the other person's shoes before forming a negative opinion or taking an action that you may regret. Remember: patience, patience, patience.

Conclusion

Take some time now, and look back through this book.

If you are a novice homeworker, you have added knowledge to your formal training. You also now have a revealing view of situations that you may encounter in your professional future.

If you were a mediocre homeworker, but still had a healthy attitude toward your clients, you have become a more understanding, more conscientious homeworker.

If you were an excellent homeworker, you now have confirmation of your skills, and perhaps you have acquired new insights about the needs you fill for a client.

If you are an advocate and have read this book, you now possess valuable information you can use to assist the client to find the best of homecare. You have acquired a clearer vision of the positive qualities and negative traits to look for in a homeworker. And you now have some idea of how to keep your sanity throughout the process.

And if you are the client and have taken the contents of this book to heart, you have accepted the necessity of having day-to-day help, developed a plan to find a homeworker compatible with you, and learned how to live with *Homecare, the Best*.

Appendix A

Sample Job Description

Position For: Certified Nurse Aide
Live-in, On-Call 24 Hours

Date June 12, 1999

Client Name   Mrs. A Beafa   Age 68
                       Spouse Warren (deceased)
Address   0000 Far Street, Apt. 222
                       Orangeade, New Jersey
Phone   (000) 000-0000
Client Advocate   Mrs. Mary Main

Client's Needs:

Mrs. Beafa was diagnosed with Parkinson's disease in May of 1996. She experiences mild tremors most of the time, with occasional episodes of a more serious nature. She walks with the support of a three-legged cane and sometimes with minimum assistance from a helper.

Mrs. Beafa has partial deafness in her left ear and wears a hearing aid during the day. Her diet as outlined by her physician is low-fat, low-cholesterol. She has no mental impairments, and she lays out and takes all medications without assistance.

Social and Personal Preferences:

Mrs. Beafa plays bridge every Thursday at her condo clubhouse and has lunch or dinner out two or three times a week with friends or relatives. She enjoys TV: "Oprah," "The Regis and Kathy Lee Show," ice hockey, and the "Channel 9 News" at six o'clock. She also likes playing gin and Scrabble. Swimming is a passion of hers, and she usually goes to the pool three or four mornings a week.

Daily Schedule:

Mrs. Beafa gets up at 7:30 and has breakfast in the kitchen at 8 o'clock. Pool visits are usually made between 9 a.m. and 11 a.m. Lunch is at noon; afternoons are spent shopping, taking care of correspondence, or making telephone calls. Mrs. Beafa may take a rest between 2:30 and 4:30. Dinner is at 6 o'clock, and Mrs. Beafa retires at 10 p.m.

Regular Duties of Nurse Aide:

Prepare light meals. Assist client with bath and personal grooming, accompany client to pool, on shopping trips, to doctor and other appointments, assist client with opening mail and making phone calls, and take part in leisure activities at home; these include playing cards and watching TV. Remind client, if necessary, when medications are to be taken.

Worker's Meal and Rest Breaks:

Breakfast at 8:45 for 30 minutes. Lunch and dinner at same times as client. Food provided by client. Rest Breaks: Two hours in the afternoon, hours to be decided during first week of employment.

Special Requests:

Feed two cockatiels daily and change paper in birdcage once a week. Occasionally, use client's car to pick up relatives at local airport. Nonsmoker, nondrinker preferred.

Current Household Staff:

Housekeeper: Ruth–two mornings per week
Yardman: Russell–two days per week
Cook: Briette–prepares lunch and dinner on weekends

Live-in Accommodations:

Bedroom and private bath

Worker Break Area:

Kitchen, pool area, or guest bedroom

Telephone Use:

Second line with worker's calling card

Vacation Periods:

One paid week after one year
Live-in worker: Additional time off to be discussed at hire

On-Job Visits with Worker by Friends and Family:

To be discussed.

Pay Rate:

Live-in 5 days, on call 24 hours—beginning pay $170 per day.
Raise considered after 12 months.

Appendix B

Additional Readings and Reference Sources

This appendix contains three kinds of resources: books, Web sites, and handwriting analysts. Many titles and association names have the word "parent" in them, but keep in mind that the practical and emotional skills used when caring for a parent can be used when giving care to any person.

Beat the Nursing Home Trap, Matthews, Joseph, Nolo Press Berkeley, Second Edition, 1995. Tells how to assess needs. Covers homecare, elder residences, nursing facilities, Medicare, Medicaid, Veterans' benefits, asset protection, long-term care, estate planning, and much more in simple and easy to understand format.

The Caregiver's Guide, Rob, Caroline, R.N., with Janet Reynolds, G.N.P., Houghton Mifflin Company, 1991. Most of this book gives information on specific diseases and how to cope with clients who have them. Chapter 15 "Help and Where to Find It," pages 342–400, is especially helpful. Overall wordy, but good information.

The Caregiver's Handbook, Visiting Nurse Association of America, DK Publishing, 1998. Contains numerous illustrations and explanations of caregiving skills and techniques. Excellent for friends and family members serving as caregivers. Also an excellent manual for professional caregivers who need to review skills of hands-on care.

The Caregiver's Manual, Williams, Gene B., and Patie Kay, Carol Publishing Group, 1995. Practical tips on caregiving. Instructions to help with decision making.

Caregiving, Horne, Jo, American Association for Retired People, 1985. Especially relevant are Chapters 1–5.

Caring for Your Aging Parents, Cohen, Donna, Ph.D., and Carl Eisdorfer, Ph.D., M.D., G.P. Putnam's Sons, 1995. Wordy but good information. Organized into seven steps that cover problems of parent care, denial, managing your emotions, caregiving partnerships, balancing needs, allocating resources, and using crisis and management skills.

Caring for Your Parents: a Sourcebook, McLean, Helene, Doubleday, 1987. Especially helpful is Chapter 5, "Helping Your Parents Make Their Way through the Health Insurance Maze," Chapter 7, "Homecare: How Everyone Benefits," and pages 235–237, which explain the role of a professional care manager.

Caring for Your Aging Parents, Smith, Kerri S., American Source Books, 1992. Small book. Easy to read. Includes schedules and timesaving tips that are especially helpful.

The Complete and Easy Guide to Social Security and Medicare 1995, Jehle, Faustin F., Fraser-Vance Publishing, 1995. Exactly what the title says it is.

Complete Eldercare Planner, Loverde, Joy, Hyperion, 1997. A practical guide. Workbook format includes checklists, question lists to use when researching, and resource names and telephone numbers.

Eldercare, What to Look For, What to Look Out For!, Cassidy, Thomas M., New Horizon Press, 1997. Good advice on how to make wise hiring decisions. Chapter 12 contains the section, "Twenty Questions Frequently Asked by Those in an Eldercare Crisis."

H & R Block 1996 Income Tax Guide, Anderson, Nance, George Corney, and Susan Van Alstyne, eds., Simon & Schuster, 1996. (Use the current version of this guide, of course.) Contains solid information on IRS tax rules governing payments to household help. Household employees usually include companions, domestics, healthcare workers, and custodial workers. Look for these terms in the index: Self-employed, Household employee, Medical expenses, Back-up withholding, Family members—as caregivers, Form 1099 MISC, and Form W-9.

The Handbook of Hospice Care, Buckingham, Robert W., Dr. P.H., Prometheus Books, 1996. Good information in easy to understand format. A lot of the information can be used in *any* caregiving and/or homecare situation.

The Hospice Choice, Lattanzi-Licht, Marcia, with John J. Mahoney and Galen W. Miller, Fireside, Simon and Schuster, 1998. Covers it all—what to expect of hospice and the wide range of services available through hospice.

How to Care for Aging Parents, Moore, Virginia, Worman Publishing Company, 1996. Wide-ranging. Touches on everything from talking about care to grieving after a parent's death. Especially helpful is "Getting Help: Community and Home Care Services," pages 166 through 189. Also gives good information on reverse mortgages.

How to Care for Your Aging Parents . . . And Still Have a Life of your Own, Dolan, Michael, Mulholland Pacific, 1992. Personal narrative, which includes practical information. Author gives a frank and realistic view of coping with a parent who can no longer manage independent living. Can be used with clients, as well. Excellent.

How to Care for Your Parents, Levin, Nora Jean, W.W. Norton & Company, 1997. Extremely practical guide to finding help on the Internet. Almost a textbook in learning to explore the myriad information fibers of the Web. More immediately helpful are pages 15-100.

J.K. Lasser's Your Income Tax, 1996, J.K. Lasser Institute, McMillan, U.S.A., 1996. Check the index for these keywords: Household employee, Independent contractor, Self-employed. On pages 378–379 of this edition, you will find good information regarding payments made to household employees. Check the latest edition for changes.

Keys to Survival for Caregivers, Kouri, Mary K., Ph.D., Barron's, 1992. A small book containing concise information. Covers "Anger and Caregiving" and "Guilt and Caregiving." Offers good information on finances, legal matters, and paperwork involved in the caregiving process.

Long Distance Caregiving, Heath, Angela, M.G.S., American Source Books, 1993. Excellent, to-the-point information on this subject.

Making the Most of Medicare, Pell, Arthur R., Ph.D., Fraser-Vance Publishing Company, 12th Edition, 1987. Ignore publishing date. Information in this book is every bit as relevant now as then. Especially helpful is "Homecare", pages 77–78. Check current information, but read "Medicare," pages 1–6, and "Medicaid," pages 59–66.

The Medicaid Planning Handbook, Bove, Alexander A., Jr., Little, Brown, and Company, 1996. Defines and outlines Medicaid plans clearly. Covers everything from protecting assets and appeals to planning for an incompetent spouse.

A Medical Handbook for Senior Citizens and Their Families, Thorton, Howard A., M.D., Auburn House Publishing, 1989. In-depth explanations about illnesses, diseases, symptoms, treatments, etc. Especially helpful is Chapter 30, pages 261–276. An excellent reference.

Medicare Made Easy, Inlander, Charles B., and Michael A. Donio, People's Medical Society, Revised and Updated Edition, 1998. Explains clearly the guidelines for Medicare homecare coverage. Includes a helpful question and answer section.

The Merck Manual, Berkow, Robert, M.D., Andrew J. Fletcher, M.B., B.Chir., Mark H. Beers, eds., Merck and Company, Inc., 16th Edition. There is also a *Merck Manual, Home Edition*, which has numerous illustrations, but the standard 16th edition is not that difficult to understand. Many doctors are hesitant to offer information that can help caregivers serve their clients with confidence. Merck books provide the layperson with disease descriptions, symptoms, diagnosis, treatments, and prognosis—information that may be helpful in caring for clients who need medical assistance. A caregiver will not "play" doctor, but with correct knowledge of a client's medical condition, one can know what to watch for and when to call for help.

The Myth of Senility, Henig, Robin Marantz, Anchor Press, Doubleday, 1981. Written in narrative style, this book will help you to understand how memory works. Especially helpful is the information given about depression, drugs, and self-help.

Old Age is not for Sissies, Linkletter, Art, Viking, 1998. Written with great warmth and insight. Especially helpful are Chapter 2, "The Right to Live Independently," Chapter 3, "Housing Choices," and Chapter 5, " Freedom from Fear of Abuse."

Simplifying Your Life As a Senior Citizen, Cleveland, Joan, St. Martin's Griffin, 1998. Easy to read information about practical aspects of homecare: driving, vision, hearing, home hazards, and much more.

The 36-Hour Day, Mace, Nancy L., and Peter V. Rabins, M.D., Warner Books, 1991. Written primarily for caregivers with clients who have Alzheimer's disease, but excellent reading for everyone. Especially helpful is Chapter 3, which gives insight into what is going on inside the client's mind. Chapter 4 covers "Problems in Independent Living," Chapter 5 enlightens on "Problems Arising in Everyday Care," and Chapter 7 lists "Problems of Behavior."

What the IRS Doesn't Want You to Know, Kaplan, Carl, CPA, and Naomi Weiss, Fourth Edition, Revised and Updated for 1998, Villard, Random House, 1997. Explains clearly the differences between independent contractors and employees, pages 156–160; explains back-up withholding on page 127.

When Your Parents Need You, Robinson, Rita, IBS Press, 1990. Excellent reading for family members serving as caregivers. Covers feelings of guilt and family relation- ships. It also gives a clear explanation of Medi-Cal, which is California's system of Medicaid.

You and Your Aging Parent, Silverstone, Barbara, and Helen Kendel Hyman, Pantheon, Third Edition, 1989. Focuses on problems of aging, but is helpful to anyone needing homecare. Especially helpful is Chapter 3, "The Family Merry-Go-Round," pages 38-58, Chapters 7 and 8, and Chapter 10, pages 239–255.

Homecare-related Web Sites

Once you access any of the following sites you will be rewarded with a plethora of information that includes referrals to homecare providers.

- Administration on Aging: **(http://www.aoa.dhhs.gov.)** Has numerous links to other sites.
- American Association of Home and Services for the Aging **(http://www.aahsa.org)**
- American Association of Retired Persons **www.aarp.org**
- The American Geriatrics Society

   (http://www.americangeriatrics.org) Good information on all areas of aging.
- Careguide **(http://www.careguide.net)** (locate Children of Aging Parents here)
- Friends Life Care at Home **(http://www.friendslifecareathome.com)**
- Home Care On-line; National Association for Home Care **(http://www.nahc.org)** Has a nonmember locator service.
- Home Instead Senior Care

   (http://www.homeinstead.com)
- Housecall Medical Resources, Inc. **(http://www.housecall.com)**
- National Association of Professional Care Managers

   (http://www.caremanager.org) Locates caremanagers across the country.
- Medicaid **(http://www.hcfa.gov)**
- Medicare **(http://www.ssa/gov)**
- U.S. Department of Veterans Affairs **(http://www.va.gov)** Information on homecare coverage provided.

- Third Age Media, Inc. (**http://www.thirdage.com/family/caregiving/tools/payoptions**)
  Good information with many helpful links.
- National Hospice (**http://www.nho.org/database.htm**)

Handwriting Analysts

Handwriting Analyst
Rodger Rubin
29 West 65th Street,
New York, NY 10023
(212) 580-9808

Handwriting Analyzed, Inc.
George Johnson
P.O. Box 165,
Sharpsville, PA 16150
(724)-962-1448

Manhattan Handwriting Consultant
Janice Klein
250 West 57th Street, Suite 1228-A
New York, NY 10107
(212) 265-1148

Write Choice
Sheila Lowe
(805) 259-8979

Appendix C

Organizations and Associations

These organizations and associations supply information and assistance to clients, advocates, and caregivers. As evidenced by their names, some render support to persons with specific diseases; others target specific problem areas. Before calling for information, write out your questions and be as specific as possible when asking them.

Alzheimer's Association
(800) 272-3900   (312) 335-8700

Cancer Care Counseling Line
(800) 813-4673

Alliance for Children and Family
(800) 221-2681

American Geriatrics Society
(800) 247-4779   (212) 308-1414

Association of Jewish Family Services
(800) 634-7346

Catholic Charities
(800) 886-4295

Children of Aging Parents
(214) 945-6900   (215) 945-6900

Eldercare Locator
(800) 677-1116

International Center for the Disabled
(212) 679-0100   (212) 585-6254
(212) 889-0372 –TTY

Internal Revenue Service
(800) 829-1040 Information
(800) 829-3676 Forms

Medicare
(800) 638-6833

National Alliance for Caregiving
(301) 718-8444

National Association of Area Agencies on Aging
(202) 296-8130

National Association of Professional Geriatric Care Managers
(520) 881-8008

National Foundation of Interfaith Volunteer
Caregivers, Inc.
(703) 243-5900   (800) 338-8619

National Health Information Center
(800) 336-4797

National Hospice Helpline
(800) 658-8898

Program of All-inclusive Care for the Elderly (PACE)
(415) 749-2680

Social Security Administration
(FHCA–Medicare/Medicaid Information)
(800) 772-1213

Veterans Administration
(800) 827-1000

Visiting Nurse Association of America—
Visiting Nurses Preferred Care
(303) 753-0218

Visiting Nurse Association–Referrals
(888) 866-8773

Appendix D

State Bureaus of Licensing, Nurse Aides

These state offices can verify the license(s) status of nurse aides, nurse assistants, and/or certified nurse aides. Many of these numbers are serviced by recorded menus, and you will be asked to make selections to obtain information. Listen carefully before you make a selection, and be ready to touch-tone the aide's social security number if asked to do so.

Alabama
  (334) 206-5169

Alaska
  (907) 561-2171

Arizona
  (602) 331-8111

Arkansas
  (501) 682-8430
  (501) 682-8484

California
  (916) 445-2070

Colorado
  (303) 894-7888

Connecticut:
  Nurse Aides
  (860) 509-7596
  Home Health Aides
  (860) 509-7400

Delaware
(302) 577-6666

District of Columbia
  (202) 726-7824

Florida
  (850) 414-7209

Georgia
  (800) 282-4579

Hawaii
  (808) 739-8122

Idaho
  (208) 334-3110

Illinois
  (217) 782-3070

Indiana
  (317) 232-2960

Iowa
  (515) 281-4115

Kansas
  (785) 296-1250

Kentucky
Charge is 2.95+.50 min
(900) 555-5700

Lousiana
(504) 925-4132

Maine
(207) 624-5205

Maryland
(410) 764-2770

Massachusetts
(617) 727-5860

Michigan
(800) 748-0252

Minnesota
(612) 617-2270

Mississippi
(601) 987-6858

Missouri
(573) 751-3082

Montana
(406) 444-4980

Nebraska
(402) 471-0537

Nevada
(702) 486-5800

New Hampshire
(603) 271-6599

New Jersey
(610) 617-9300

New Mexico
(505) 827-4200

New York
(800) 274-7181

North Carolina
Nurse Aide
(919) 733-2786
Nurse Aide II
(919) 881-2272

North Dakota
Nurse Aide
(701) 328-2388
Reg. Nurse Aide
(701) 328-9780

Ohio
(614) 752-9522

Oklahoma
(405) 271-4085

Oregon
(503) 731-3459

Pennsylvania
(717) 783-6965

Puerto Rico
(787) 725-8161

Rhode Island
(401) 222-2827

South Carolina
(800) 475-8290

South Dakota
(605) 362-2760

Tennessee
Long menu. Ignore "access code"
and touch-tone 2222 when asked
(615) 741-7670

Texas
(800) 452-3934

Utah
(801) 530-6628

Vermont
(802) 828-2453
(802) 828-2396

Virgin Islands
(340) 776-7397

Virginia
(804) 662-7636
(804) 662-9909

Washington
(360) 664-4111
(360) 236-4702

West Virginia
(304) 558-0688

Wisconsin
(608) 267-2374

Wyoming
(307) 777-7601

Appendix E

State Listings of Area Agencies on Aging

Calling these Area Agency on Aging state offices, you will get a referral number to an office in the county in which you reside. The county office can offer you referrals to sources in your area for homecare information.

Alabama
(334) 242-5743

Alaska
(907) 465-4879

Arizona
(602) 542-4446

Arkansas
(501) 682-2441

California
(916) 322-5290

Colorado
(303) 620-4147

Connecticut
(860) 424-5277

Delaware
(302) 577-4791

District of Columbia
(202) 724-5622

Florida
(850) 414-2000

Georgia
(404) 657-5258

Hawaii
(808) 586-0100

Idaho
(208) 334-2423

Illinois
(217) 785-2870

Indiana
(317) 232-7020

Iowa
(515) 281-5187

Kansas
(785) 296-4986

Kentucky
(502) 564-6930

Louisiana
(225) 342-7100

Maine
(207) 624-5335

Maryland
(410) 767-1100

Massachusetts
(617) 222-7470

Michigan
(517) 373-8230

Minnesota
(651) 296-2770

Mississippi
(601) 359-4929

Missouri
(573) 751-3082

Montana
(406) 444-7788

Nebraska
(402) 471-2307

Nevada
(702) 486-3545

New Hampshire
(603) 271-4394

New Jersey
(609) 588-3601

New Mexico
(505) 827-7640

New York
(518) 474-5731

North Carolina
(919) 733-3983

North Dakota
(701) 328-8909

Ohio
(614) 466-5500

Oklahoma
(405) 521-2327

Oregon
(503) 945-5811

Pennsylvania
(717) 783-1550

Puerto Rico
(787) 721-5710

Rhode Island
(401) 222-2858

South Carolina
(803) 253-6177

South Dakota
(605) 773-3656

Tennessee
(615) 741-2056

Texas
(512) 424-6840

Utah
(801) 538-3910

Vermont
(802) 241-2400

Virginia
(804) 662-9333

Virgin Islands
(340) 692-5950

Washington
(360) 902-7797

West Virginia
(304) 558-3317

Wisconsin
(608) 266-2536

Wyoming
(307) 777-7986

Index

About the Author

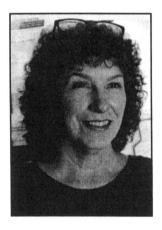

Jo Whatley Cheatham has spent most of her professional life giving care and smoothing out turmoil as a healthcare worker—not only for paying clients, but for many friends and family members as well. Jo attended colleges in North Carolina and Alabama. She is now a Florida licensed certified nurse assistant (CNA), and in that capacity, has worked with numerous clients, their friends and families, healthcare and staffing agencies, and countless domestic and healthcare workers. When it comes to homecare, she has "been there, done that."

In 1991 Jo started ProblemSolvers, a consumer advocacy and information brokering company through which she schedules lectures on homecare and caregiving. In her spare time, Jo studies graphology, reads *Cecil Textbook of Medicine,* and tends the ailing plants on her patio.

The author invites and welcomes all comments, questions, and/or personal experience-sharing from readers and will be pleased to schedule a lecture on homecare. You may reach her as follows:

Jo Cheatham
ProblemSolvers: (407) 783-1888
P.O. Box 320610
Cocoa Beach, FL 32931

www.problemsolvers8.xtcom.com
(Contains E-mail link)

ORDER FORM

Order by
Fax: (407) 868-4684
Mail: ProSo Press
      P.O. Box 320610
      Cocoa Beach, FL   32932-0610

Or call toll free: 1-888-783-3912
*Call or write for bulk order prices and shipping charges
Permanent mailing address:
Name: _____

Address: _____

City: _____

State: _____ Zip: _____

Telephone: _____

HOMECARE: *The Best!* Price per copy: 14.95
Number of copies: _____ @ 14.95 each   Total $_____
Shipping:$ 3.00 one copy, $1.50 each add'nl copy $_____
                         Subtotal $_____
Sales tax: Florida residents add 6% tax $_____

                       Total amount $_____

Method of payment:
__Check/Money Order __ MasterCard __ Am. Express __Visa
Credit card number:_____

Expiration date:_____

Name on card (Please *write*)
_____